AVELINE

Dear Aey & Jan

I pray for you

Happy life!!

文月信子

April 27, 1997

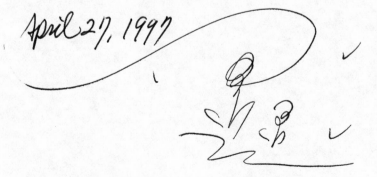

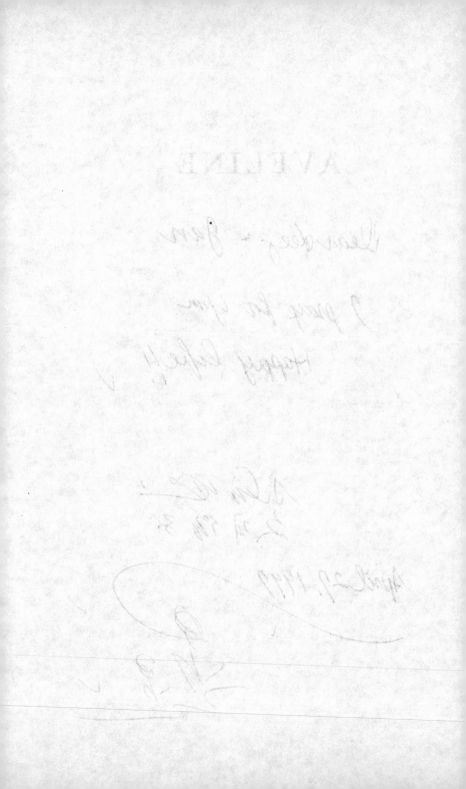

AVELINE

The Life and Dream
of the Woman Behind
Macrobiotics Today

By Aveline Kushi
with Alex Jack

Foreword by Michio Kushi

Japan Publications, Inc.

Published by JAPAN PUBLICATIONS, INC., Tokyo & New York

Distributors:
UNITED STATES: *Kodansha International/USA, Ltd., through Harper & Row, Publishers, Inc., 10 East 53rd Street, New York, N. Y. 10022.*
SOUTH AMERICA: *Harper & Row, Publishers, Inc., International Department.* CANADA: *Fitzhenry & Whiteside Ltd., 195 Allstate Parkway, Markham, Ontario, L3R 4T8.* MEXICO & CENTRAL AMERICA: *HARLA S. A. de C. V. Apartado 30–546, Mexico 4, D. F.*
BRITISH ISLES: *Premier Book Marketing Ltd., 1 Gower Street, London WC1E 6HA.* EUROPEAN CONTINENT (except Germany): *PBD Proost & Brandt Distribution bv, Strijkviertel 63, 3454 PK de Meern, The Netherlands.* GERMANY: *PBV Proost & Brandt Verlagsauslieferung, Herzstrasse 1, 5000 Köln 40, Germany.*
AUSTRALIA & NEW ZEALAND: *Bookwise International, 1 Jeanes Street, Beverley, South Australia 5007.* THE FAR EAST & JAPAN: *Japan Publications Trading Co., Ltd., 1–2–1, Sarugaku-cho, Chiyoda-ku, Tokyo 101.*

First edition: April 1988
LCCC No. 87–080492
ISBN 0–87040–693–0

Printed in Japan

Foreword

MARRIAGE is one of the loveliest blossoms of the unfolding spiral of life. It involves encountering all aspects of human nature—sensory and emotional, intellectual and economical, social and philosophical, spiritual and sometimes cosmological. In some instances, the husband leads and the wife follows; in other instances, the wife leads and the husband follows. However, true marriage rests on two fundamental grounds: 1) biological similarity—eating the same or similar food—and, 2) similarity or oneness in cosmological and spiritual vision—sharing the same purpose and dream in life. These two essential conditions, biological and spiritual, become the constitution for holding, carrying forward, and realizing married life together, especially after children are born.

I constantly marvel that Aveline has so faithfully observed proper dietary practice since the time I first saw her in New York in 1951. For nearly forty years, she has been the anchor for the whole family in a sea of swirling currents. On this biological foundation, she has maintained her own health in addition to that of her husband and children. Because of her natural discipline in preparing nourishing whole foods with a calm, peaceful mind, no family member has experienced any serious sickness in nearly half a century. I admire her resolve and am grateful to her understanding and practice in this essential aspect of life.

I have also been continuously impressed with Aveline's sense of righteousness. From time to time, she might have expressed stubbornness, impatience, rigidity, and miscommunication toward family or friends. However, regardless of how her expression might have appeared, her underlying motive has always been a clear sense of righteousness—righteousness not in the usual ethical sense, but the righteousness of humanity living on this planet according to the natural law of the universe. Her sense of righteousness has often taken the form of self-reflection concerning the behavior of other family members and friends. No wonder she has been seeking her own cultural refinement and seeking more meditative spiritual realization. She has demonstrated this quest in deepening her mastery of the tea ceremony, flower arrangement, and Noh dance, as well as in cooking. Furthermore, she has shown her serious practice in meditation, chanting, and prayers related primarily to Buddhism, Christianity, and Shintoism but not limited only to them. She even periodically practices chanting ten thousand times every morning for one hundred days.

In bringing up our children, Aveline did not act as the usual mother in modern society. She did not encourage them to be academically competitive in high school or college, but she has constantly concerned herself with their physical health, psychological well-being, and clear thinking and direction in life. Uppermost in her mind has been whether they are doing what they really wish to do and whether their actions and visions are related to the benefit of society and eventually the world. The standard of success that she expects is not valued by the amount of income attained or by the occupational position reached. Instead, her measure of success is more directly related to human nature—the development of each child's health, character, behavior, vision, and endless dream to pursue what he or she wants and can contribute to human society as a whole. I sincerely hope that our children and grandchildren will understand and comprehend what their mother and grandmother has continuously prayed for them to realize.

Though her expression often appears to be serious, Aveline has retained through the years, to my frequent surprise, a childlike instinct and manner. This playful nature has often been demonstrated without her apparent knowledge, for example, when she dances with her young students, runs on the street, converses on the phone, and expresses her views in meetings of various kinds. Beyond her immediate family, Aveline has also maintained her love and care for thousands of people, especially young people with whom she has the opportunity to meet often. All these years she has kept by her side the beautiful poems that her grammar school students wrote when she first taught school in the deep mountains of Japan over forty years ago. Several years ago she edited and published their verses and sent a copy to each student. By then, most of them were already parents with school age children of their own. I have also been impressed with the love, care, and closeness Aveline shares with relatives, friends, and acquaintances. Recently, we visited the village where she was born and grew up, in Yokota, and I was amazed at the warm reception she received from her former students, teachers, neighbors, and fellow villagers. All of them expressed their fondness for Aveline and gathered around her, spending days and nights together chatting about old times, exchanging snapshots of children and grandchildren, and eating wild mountain grasses and other delicacies for which that part of Izumo province has long been renowned.

Many people comment how graceful Aveline is when she teaches cooking or cultural arts. It is impressive to see the natural gracefulness in her movement as she handles grains and vegetables, pots and pans, and pens and brushes; when she wears a kimono, sari, or party dress; and when she performs Japanese spiritual practices, writes letters, and does calligraphy. On these occasions, people are impressed that her naturally graceful movement has no excess. It appears as water gently streaming down or a spring wind breezing by.

During our married life, I often wondered why Aveline and I came together to share this lifetime, having children and devoting ourselves to realizing the same vision. There have been many factors bringing us together, including the similar social background of growing up during wartime, the same vision of creating a world of enduring peace through macrobiotics, the study with a common teacher, George Ohsawa,

and our arrival in America fairly soon after World War II.
But still, from time to time, I wondered whether there was
some deeper connection. Then it recently became clear when
I visited her native area in Izumo province. Since mythological
times, her town, Yokota, has been known as the home of
Kushi-Inada-Hime (the Wondrous Princess of the Rice Fields).
An hour's drive from this town, on the Sea of Japan, is
the Kumano Grand Shrine. Dedicated to Kushi-Mike-No
(Wondrous God and Goddess of Food and Way of Life), this
shrine is connected with Kumano-Hongu, the central shrine
in Kumano, in Wakayama, my family's native town and province in southern Japan.

It is this spiritual destiny for which we came together. Our
life has been devoted to sharing the same dream of teaching
and spreading proper dietary practice and way of life in order
to prevent and reverse the wave of degenerative disease and
the threat of war that is enveloping the world and to ensure
humanity's continued biological and spiritual evolution. Human
life is ephemeral. Human affairs are more ephemeral. Inevitably the time will come for us to depart from each other or
separate, but I know that our dream and vision are insepar-
able and everlasting. So long as the human race continues to
live on this planet, our dream of a unified, healthy, peaceful
world will not perish.

I extend my sincere gratitude to Aveline. On this occasion,
the publication of her autobiography, I wish to celebrate the
achievements that she has made by herself, through me,
together with me, and together with many friends. Many
people may not yet be aware, but because of her, America,
Europe, eventually Japan and Africa, as well as other parts of
the world, will become healthier and happier and move closer
toward realizing one peaceful world.

I further extend my gratitude to Alex Jack who has been
studying with me for many years. He has contributed to
deepening our thought in writing several of my books. Without him, *Aveline: The Life and Dream of the Woman Behind
Macrobiotics Today* would not have been possible. Without

his visit to Japan to learn about Aveline's background, readers of this book would not find so many delicate threads and patterns that have been woven together to tell the story of her life. Many people do not know that woman is the force opening the door to human health, freedom, peace, and happiness.

I also wish to express my sincere thanks to the publisher, Japan Publications, Inc., for their dedication to the cause of serving world society and their steady encouragement and wholehearted support in bringing out this book. I pray that Aveline's life, dream, and spirit will continue to inspire and touch the hearts of people the world over for endless generations to come.

MICHIO KUSHI
August 29, 1987
Brookline, Massachusetts

Preface

"Human laws must emphasize the decrees of nature."
—Samuel Butler, *Erewhon*.

I N THE BEGINNING, AIDS appeared out of nowhere. Like
a ferocious dragon, it laid waste the countryside. First it
devoured the weak, the unattached, people from distant
lands, and those generally at the bottom of society. But soon
AIDS moved into the capital and started consuming the strong
and powerful. It struck alike the pious and the impious, rich
and poor, female and male, old and young. The new plague
left everyone frightened. Some hospitals refused admittance to
people with AIDS, and many doctors and nurses wouldn't treat
them or insisted on wearing rubber gloves. Landlords evicted
them from their apartments. Ministers denied them use of
churches, chapels, and communion cups. Restaurants refused
them service. Spouses, partners, parents, and children aban-
doned them.

My husband is ordinarily a very patient person. Outside of
his usual teaching and counseling activities, he is content sitting
in the coffee shop, drawing spirals on his napkin, and watching
the world go by. Almost nothing upsets him. Behind every
difficulty, he sees a blessing and opportunity for self-reflection.
But in the case of AIDS, he became very angry. He could not
bear to see people treated as lepers and outcasts. He vowed
to free society of this terrible scourge, which was affecting the
mind and spirit worse than the body.

We went to New York City to work with people with
AIDS. New York was the capital of the epidemic. We had
lived near Columbia University and in Queens twenty years
earlier. We still visited Manhattan several times a year to

give lectures and macrobiotic cooking classes.

The meetings were held in Greenwich Village. My first impression was one of darkness and depression. The young men who gathered couldn't hold their heads up. They were sad and without hope. The surroundings were also bleak.

My husband talked to them about macrobiotics. He told them that AIDS was caused by a longtime imbalance in their way of eating. "The basic cause of AIDS is ignorance of health, especially the power of daily food. Other features of modern life have contributed to the weakening or lowering of our natural immunity. These include lack of breastfeeding as babies, childhood immunizations, tonsillectomies and other harmful or unnecessary operations, and use of prescription and recreational drugs. A virus might transmit the disease, but it is the agent rather than the underlying cause of the problem. Unless our blood quality is already weakened by years of eating meat and sugar, dairy food and tropical fruit, and ice cream and soft drinks and by too much medical intervention and drug abuse, the virus cannot secure a foothold in our body."

He said that with proper cooking, it was possible to reverse AIDS. The men had never heard such things before. They had been told their condition was invariably fatal. At most they could hope to receive an experimental drug that might ease their dying pain.

But even more remarkable was the way my husband interacted with the young friends with AIDS. He shook their hands, clasped their shoulders, and embraced them. He did not wash his hands after being with them. They were astonished. Even the most compassionate doctors and clergy always excused themselves to wash up and avoid contamination.

Michio also cut through the whole moral issue. Even many AIDS people themselves had secretly come to believe that they were being punished for their way of life. He reassured them that AIDS was not a moral or spiritual disease. "Society tries to change the symptoms of AIDS without changing the

underlying causes. Modern medicine tries to destroy the
disease by violent means. Religion tries to do it by eradicating
sin. This view of life is similar to fighting a war.

"There are no enemies in this universe," he continued.
"Nature brings us sickness when we ignore her laws. Harmony
is always going on between our internal and external environments. Sickness is a wonderful adjustment mechanism and a
way to localize imbalance in one part or region of the body
and allow life to continue relatively normally as a whole. By
changing our way of eating and adopting a more natural way
of life, we can restore our health and happiness. AIDS is a
disease of modern civilization. Everyone is responsible."

My husband smiled throughout his talk and tried to cheer
them up. But watching them, I was doubtful. The total atmosphere resembled young plants dying. I felt no hope.

But after we came back to New York the second time,
something changed. I didn't know why, but the feeling among
the group was much lighter. Their faces had completely
changed. The men held their heads up. Their eyes shone.
They found that joy and hope could be as contagious as fear
and suspicion. It was a great transformation. I thought too
that perhaps now I was more familiar and accepting of them.

In Soho one of our macrobiotic lady friends lent us her
beautiful studio and kitchen to give cooking classes. Soon fifty
young friends with AIDS were coming. I showed them how
to pressure-cook brown rice and make strong *miso* soup. I
showed them how to cut vegetables and soak seaweed. I went
over the basics just as I have a thousand times before in
macrobiotic cooking classes all over the world.

In class some AIDS friends started to cry. Tears of joy came
down their cheeks as we talked, touched, and ate together.
The men shared with me their sufferings, hopes, and dreams.
I was very impressed with their courage and warm sensitivity.
I was encouraged so much by their warm energy.

One of the AIDS friends from New York came up to
Boston to study at the Kushi Institute. His name was Richard.
He stayed in our home. He was an interior decorator and

entirely rearranged our house in Brookline. He was a wonderful young gentleman and enjoyed his stay with us. After completing his studies, he returned to New York and visited Texas. His legs started swelling as a result of a wider diet. We knew his condition was weak. A year later, when we were teaching in Switzerland, he called me. "I'm always thinking of you," he said in a soft, weak voice. A few days later, he passed away. I felt so sorry we couldn't help. I can still hear his clear, beautiful voice. He is with us in spirit.

AIDS is created by modern civilization's ignorance of health and human life. We all have the responsibility to change many, many things. I feel really sorry for everyone who has suffered from AIDS and other degenerative diseases.

Some medical researchers from Boston University and the Fashion Institute in New York heard about our efforts and began testing the men. Month after month, year after year, the AIDS friends patiently gave blood samples to the doctors for their study. The doctors were amazed. Some, like Richard, passed away. But on the whole the macrobiotic men continued to stabilize, and their natural immunity started to return. This was unheard of. No one before had ever survived this dread disease. The doctors began writing up their findings in important medical journals such as *The Lancet* in London and reported on their research at the International AIDS Conference in Paris. After three years, the macrobiotic AIDS friends had outlived all other AIDS patients under study. According to their psychological evaluations, they also had healthier mental outlooks and better family relations.

Many obstacles remain until society recognizes the macrobiotic solution to AIDS. Scientists are still searching for a chemical vaccine and experimenting with Star Wars-like lasers to destroy the virus. But the sharpest, most powerful weapons that modern technology has devised have proved useless in this crisis. It is hard for many people to believe that something so gentle as brown rice, miso soup, and freshly cooked vegetables and seaweed can slay the dragon of AIDS.

Also it is very difficult for many of the AIDS friends to

cook for themselves or find someone knowledgeable to cook for them. My husband and I wanted to set up some institutional facility where they could come for proper cooking and guidance. In Massachusetts, my son and I went around to many hospitals, churches, and other institutions pleading for someone to lend or rent us a facility.

Everyone was very gracious. They told us, "We sympathize very much and would like to let you use our space. But the board of directors, the congregation, or the neighbors wouldn't approve."

Sooner or later, such a facility will become available. In the case of heart disease and cancer, it took us many years to get our message across. For decades, the medical and scientific associations dismissed us as food faddists and quacks. But now they have all accepted our basic approach and issued their own dietary guidelines in essentially a macrobiotic direction. In the beginning, they wouldn't let my husband teach about diet, and now they are adopting his methods.

Every year thousands of people come to us for dietary and way of life study. A number of them are doctors and medical specialists themselves suffering from cancer, heart disease, diabetes, or arthritis. There have also been many famous people—movie stars, ambassadors, governors, senators, archbishops, a member of the president's family—who have come to our home for help.

However proud or humble, to all who come, Michio tells them the same thing, "You have created your own tumor or sickness because of what you have eaten all these years. But what you have made, you can unmake. Please follow what your grandparents, ancestors, and past generations of human beings have eaten for thousands of years. They ate principally whole grains and cooked vegetables, don't you agree? Macrobiotics is the application of traditional values and principles of natural order to daily life and consciousness in the modern world. It is nothing but common sense, intuition, or what you may call listening to the voice of God."

During our life in America, we have seen so many changes.

When we first arrived in this beautiful country over three decades ago, there was almost no good food. We discovered that we couldn't depend on the food industry, the government, or the medical profession to change. We would have to make wonderful food available to everybody ourselves. With our students and friends who shared a common dream, we convinced farmers to start growing organic brown rice and other high quality grains, beans, seeds, vegetables, and fruits. We encouraged people to eat traditionally made miso, *tamari* soy sauce, sea salt, *tofu*, *tempeh*, sea vegetables, whole-grain bread, and dozens of other healthy foods. Today the natural foods movement is world wide.

The center of our educational activities for the last twenty years has been in Boston. Doctors and scientists at the Harvard Medical School, the Framingham Heart Study, and New England Medical Center have studied the macrobiotic dietary approach and reported on its healthy benefits. In the beginning they were worried about babies and children receiving enough protein, vitamins, and other nutrients if they were not fed cow's milk, beef, chicken, eggs, and other animal foods. The researchers soon discovered that most macrobiotic children received abundant nutrients. They also were brighter and had higher IQs than ordinary children. Later the studies shifted toward heart disease and found that macrobiotic people had the lowest serum cholesterol levels and most ideal blood pressure values of any group ever tested in modern society. The studies caused a sensation and helped popularize a low-fat, high-fiber diet.

One of the oldest hospitals in Boston is the Lemuel Shattuck Hospital. It is where the nation's public health care system began nearly two hundred years ago. Several years ago, as a result of these studies, the Shattuck Hospital began serving macrobiotic food in its staff cafeteria for doctors, nurses, and other employees. Other hospitals, schools, nursing homes, and institutions have also begun serving whole foods. In Boston, the local Howard Johnson's in Kenmore Square serves miso soup and brown rice for breakfast for the many friends from around the country who come to our programs and use their facilities. In Virginia, a prison director who studied at the Kushi Institute removed sugar from his juvenile detention center, and the rate of infractions and aggressive behavior plunged by one half. Since then, macrobiotic food has begun to be introduced in other prisons around the state.

In New York, there is a macrobiotic society at the United Nations. Nearly one thousand delegates, staff, and administrators signed a petition to make macrobiotic food available in the U.N. cafeteria. In Geneva, we have been invited to teach at the World Health Organization, and there are Kushi Institutes in many of the major European capitals. In the Middle East, Central and Latin America, and other areas of conflict, macrobiotic friends have started organic farming and natural foods distribution projects to bring together warring parties, religions, and sects. In Africa, the government of the Congo has invited us to set up a program to prevent and relieve AIDS.

Several million people around the world are practicing macrobiotics today. A practical solution to the age-old problems of war, poverty, and disease is at hand. The macrobiotic way of life also offers a healthy, harmonious alternative to environmental destruction, industrial pollution, genetic engineering, and other features of modern life that challenge humanity's continued biological and spiritual evolution. My husband and I have been privileged to be part of this revolution. It is a peaceful revolution that is seeing the whole world change.

In Japan there is a wonderful children's story called *Taro Urashima*. It is about a child who visits an underground ocean empire and meets a big turtle. The turtle guides him through the invisible realm of wonder and enchantment. A few days pass, and they experience many delightful adventures. When the young hero returns to the ordinary world, he finds to his surprise that a hundred years have gone by.

I feel very much like the child in this fairy tale. From my homeland in the deep mountains of central Japan, I have been transplanted to the center of the modern world. I have seen and experienced things I never dreamed existed when growing up. My life has sped by like an arrow.

Growing up in America, my children often asked me about Japan. Many times in lectures and women's discussions, my students inquired about my background and how I came to this country. I would tell them stories about my parents, ancestors, and the small mountain village where I grew up. I recounted my own life-and-death sickness after the end of World War II and how I came to meet George Ohsawa in Tokyo and study macrobiotics. I told them of my dream for world peace and international understanding between East and West and how I sold my beautiful kimono and with the wonderful help of Mr. Shimizu came to America without a penny in my pocket. I told them how I first met my husband in the Greyhound Bus Station in Manhattan, of our immigration problems, and about our struggles to make a living and raise a family over the next ten years while laying the foundation for our future educational activities.

Over the years, I have been known by a number of names and nicknames: Koko-chan, Tomoko, Tenba, Jōtaro, Asta, and Masakari. There is an amusing tale behind each one which I tell in the chapters that follow. But the name by which I am known best is Aveline. This book is about my own journey to happiness and wholeness and my dream of a world of health and peace.

During the last thirty-five years, I have tried to live up to Aveline, my seventh and last name, and its spirit of love and compassion. I have not always succeeded and wish to apologize to my elders and teachers, my husband and family, and my students and friends for my many failures and shortcomings. For you, the reader who knows me only through these pages, I hope that my story inspires you to join our peaceful revolution and follow your own namesake or star wherever it leads you. I pray that your endless journey along the river of life is as beautiful and joyful as mine.

AVELINE KUSHI
May, 1987
Becket, Massachusetts

Contents

Foreword by Michio Kushi, 5
Preface, 11

1. By the Side of the Rice Field, 21
2. Adventures of a Heavenly Horse, 29
3. Lessons of a Peasant Sage, 41
4. Memories of Clouds Passing By, 57
5. Life at Maison Ignoramus, 91
6. The Samurai of Shinjuku Station, 115
7. Journey across the Eastern Sea, 135
8. Life in the West, 165
9. The Sprouting of American Macrobiotics, 183
10. East West Teachings and Travels, 205
11. Erewhon Lost, 231
12. The Spirit of Family Harmony, 249
13. Dancing on an Empty Stage, 271
14. Planting the Seeds of Peace, 297
15. An Obi Floating in a Stream, 311

Macrobiotic Resources, 331

1: By the Side of the Rice Field

> The many-fenced palace of Izumo
> Of the many clouds rising—
> To dwell there with my spouse
> Do I build a many-fenced palace:
> Ah, that many-fenced palace!
> —*Kojiki*

IN JAPANESE, *dō* or *tō* (Chinese: tao) means "way" and *shin* means "gods." Shintō means "Way of the Gods," and the ancient name for Japan was Shinkoku, or "Land of the Gods." The most sacred region of Japan lies in the southwest province of Izumo. Here, Izanagi and Izanami, the first parents, are said to have descended to earth from heaven and created numerous islands and offspring. After giving birth to the fire-deity, Izanami died and was buried on the border of Izumo. Her husband, Izanagi, pursued her to the next world but was unable to bring her back to life. Returning to earth, Izanagi fashioned Amaterasu, the Sun Goddess, from his left eye and Susa-no-wo, the Wind God, from his nostrils.

These events are recorded in the *Kojiki*, or "Record of Ancient Matters," Japan's oldest book. The creation of rice, millet, *azuki* beans, wheat, and soybeans is also described in this Shintō chronicle, in addition to the story of how peace came to the land. It happened in this way.

One day Susa-no-wo, the impetuous Wind God, descended from heaven to a place at the headwaters of the Hi River in the land of Izumo. Noticing some chopsticks floating in the stream, he realized the region was inhabited and came upon an old man and an old woman crying. They told him that over the years they had lost seven of their eight daughters to the

fearsome eight-headed dragon of the mountain and now the
beast was coming to claim their last child, Kushi-Inada-Hime.
Susa-no-wo promised to rescue the girl in exchange for her
hand in marriage. The parents readily consented.

Fashioning a wooden platform surrounded by eight barrels,
Susa-no-wo instructed the old man and woman to fill the
barrels with strong *sake* and wait. Soon the eight-headed
dragon came down the mountain and saw the reflection of
the girl, who was standing on the central platform, in each
barrel. Sipping rice wine from the eight barrels, the creature
soon lay down drunk. Susa-no-wo slew the sleeping serpent,
and the River Hi ran red with its blood. In its middle tail,
he found a magical sword which he presented to his sister,
the Sun Goddess. She later gave it to the ancestor of the first
emperor and, along with the sacred mirror and jewel, it became one of the three treasures of Japan. Susa-no-wo, the
culture hero of ancient Shinkoku, settled down with his bride,
Kushi-Inada-Hime, whose name means "Wondrous Princess of
the Rice Fields," and composed the song at the start of this
chapter. It is traditionally considered to be Japan's oldest
poem.

Like many Japanese children, I grew up amid these myths
and legends. But for me they had a special meaning. I was
born in Izumo province and lived in Yokota, the small mountain village where Princess Kushi-Inada-Hime was rescued
from the dragon and betrothed to Susa-no-wo.

Yokota means "By the Side of the Rice Field." The valley
in which our village was situated was very beautiful. Steep
peaks jutted up in every direction. Paddy fields and terraced
slopes extended to the foothills of the higher ranges, including
the mountain where the dragon was once said to live. Tall
evergreens dominated the forests. The surrounding woods
also contained a variety of oaks, maples, and ginkgos which
turned lovely red, silver, and gold in the autumn. Stands of
bamboo provided quilt-like patches of light green and yellow.
A narrow ribbon of highway, following the course of the Hi
River, wound through the peaks. From Yokota toward the Sea

of Japan the dusty road extended beyond the San-Yin, or Yin Mountains, about 100 miles north to Matsue, the capital of Izumo. To the south, beyond the San-Yō, or Yang Mountains, the road bore travelers about the same distance between Izumo and Hiroshima, capital of the next province.

From time immemorial, Izumo and Kyoto, to the southeast, enjoyed a very high culture. However, the peaceful, ancient agricultural society was disrupted in the 7th century B.C. when invading tribes crossed the Korean peninsula and established a new dynasty. The simple Japanese rice farmers and fishermen were no match for the invading warriors and their horses, led by the ancestor of the current emperor. They had never seen such sharp weapons and strange animals before.

By the time the *Kojiki* was written down, in the early eighth century, Izumo once again had become a sleepy agricultural province. In addition to its rice and sake—strong enough to quell a dragon's fire—Yokota was renowned for the manufacture of abacuses, traditional counting devices made of strung wooden beads. They were exported from the coastal cities, Mastue and Hamada, across the Sea of Japan, to China and Korea, besides being distributed throughout Japan.

During the middle ages, the nation was wracked by civil wars. Clan rivalries and intrigue among the shōguns spilled over from Osaka, Kyoto, and Edo into the countryside. A castle was built on the top of a prominent ridge overlooking Yokota. The village was a samurai town in those days, dotted with many Buddhist temples and Shintō shrines. In a famous battle about four hundred and fifty years ago, the castle was destroyed, with only a few ruins left to mark its site. During this period, iron manufacture increased. Since discovery of the divine sword in the dragon's tail, the surrounding mountains have been prized for their high quality iron. Among samurai, swords from Yokota became famous for their strength and durability.

Contact with the West began in the sixteenth century with the arrival of Dutch, Portuguese, and English sailors. Christian missionaries who accompanied them attracted flocks of adherents weary of the civil wars. Alarmed at the Europeans' superior firepower and religious conversions, the Tokugawa Shōgun soon closed the country to foreign influence except for a small trading post in Nagasaki. Two and a half centuries later, in 1853, Commodore Matthew G. Perry arrived with gunships from the U.S. fleet and reopened Japan to the West. The Meiji Restoration of 1868 ended the feudal era and ushered Japan into the modern age. Within a few years, the new government in Tokyo sent missions to the United States and Europe to assess Western technology. Japan quickly adopted the German medical and educational systems. A parliamentary constitution was drafted. Technical and managerial skills became valued. The samurai class that had ruled for centuries fell into disrepute, and their lands were confiscated by imperial decree.

One of the consmopolitan personalities of this era was Jō Niijima. Born and raised in Kyoto, Jō stowed away on the *Wild Rover*, a ship bound for Shanghai. Befriended by Alpheus Hardy, the owner of the vessel, the young boy eventually sailed from China to the United States. In Boston, Jō attended theological school under Hardy's auspicies, returning to Japan in the eighth year of the Meiji era.

In Edo—now Tokyo—Jō received support from Kaishu Katsu, the chief general of the last Shōgun, and from Takamori Saigo, commander of the Imperial armies who negotiated the peace treaty which resulted in the transfer of power to the young emperor and lifting of the centuries' old edict against foreign religions. The military leaders asked Jō how long he needed to build a theological school, and he replied two hundred years. Impressed with his answer, they lent him support, and in Kyoto he started Dōshisha, a Christian university that became the sister college of Amherst College in western Massachusetts. Jō later served as a guide and translator for one of the Japanese embassies visiting the West, and following his death General Katsu wrote a famous inscription on his grave.

Among the Christian sects that flourished in the latter part of the nineteenth century was the Salvation Army. Founded by William and Catherine Booth amid the squalor of Victorian London, the Salvation Army saw its mission as spreading the word of the Lord and feeding and caring for the poor and oppressed. Within several decades, its chapters crisscrossed the world. The Salvation Army's militant service to God and society especially appealed to Japan's former samurai class imbued with the Bushido spirit. Booth himself was a vegetarian, though diet did not figure in the church's teachings.

Gunpei Yamamuro, founder of the Japanese Salvation Army, enlisted the support of Mr. Okazaki, a young theological student at Dōshisha University. Okazaki brought Booth's gospel of enlistment in the Army of God back to his home village. Yokota at that time numbered about two hundred homes. In 1915, Okazaki and his small band of supporters sang songs and beat a big drum at a festival in Yokota to attract followers. According to a contemporary newspaper account, "Corps Sergeant-Major Okazaki played the drum in blood and fire style," and there was speculation that "surely Okazaki has gone mad." However, the farmers responded to his sincerity. Within a short time he recruited fifty members and set up a clinic, day nursery, and sewing club. Later that year, Mr. Okazaki visited San Francisco, meeting relatives, talking with church leaders in the United States, and inspecting the postal system for which he worked back home. Upon his return, he started a women's college in Yokota which he named Respecting Love. He felt that women's education was very important for Japan's future. For far too long, girls and women had been confined in ignorance of the larger world.

Meanwhile, a young medical doctor, Akio Fujiwara, returned to Yokota from medical college, built a hospital, and became a pillar of the church. After centuries, practitioners of traditional Oriental medicine had lost sight of the underlying principles of yin and yang. Dietary guidelines and folk remedies had degenerated into fixed codes and magical elixirs which offered little relief to the spread of tuberculosis, smallpox, and other infectious diseases.

In the turbulent period following the end of the feudal era, the economic, social, and cultural upheavals that engulfed Japan must have seemed like the reawakening of the great eight-headed dragon. Though the Salvationists were initially viewed with alarm, their good will and perseverance eventually brought social change and recognition. In Tokyo, after braving pitched battles in the streets, church leaders succeeded in liberating tens of thousands of young women—mostly indentured farm girls, not unlike Princess Kushi-Inada-Hime's hapless sisters—from brothels. In 1920 the nation officially honored five Westerners who had come to the country since the beginning of the Meiji era as benefactors of Japan. Two were leaders of the Salvation Army. Also twice the Emperor decorated Colonel Yamamuro for his work to free the poor and destitute.

Among the staunch local followers of the new religion in Yokota was Banjiro Yokoyama. Descendent of rural samurai, Yokoyama grew up in impoverished circumstances. His father, a building contractor, had built the local schoolhouse but lost his wealth because of a set contract that did not cover anticipated expenses. His mother died shortly after his birth. At an early age, he went to Kyoto to learn the silkscreen trade so that he would prosper. As a teenager, Yokoyama enrolled in Bible classes and became a devout Christian. Influenced by Mr. Okazaki and Dr. Fujiwara, he decided not to smoke or drink sake. When he was drafted into the army, Yokoyama arrived carrying a Bible and wearing a kimono and Salvation Army hat. The officers sent him to jail. But he remained determined and wouldn't part with the gospel and uniform. Recognizing his iron will, the authorities permitted him to rejoin his unit.

Upon returning to Yokota, Yokoyama began working for Dr. Fujiwara and started thinking about marriage and raising a family. The village doctor thought that Katsue, an earnest young woman who was born into a farm family in the next village and became a Catholic as a teenager, might make a suitable match. He felt Katsue's practical, down-to-earth nature, love of children, and wonderful cooking skills would perfectly complement the impetuous but hardworking young artisan. The doctor introduced the young pair, and the couple's wedding—accompanied by traditional gifts of sticky *mochi*, or pounded sweet rice, symbolic of staying together— marked the first Christian betrothal in this region of Izumo.

In this way, my parents came to be united. I was born the same spring that Yokota's Salvation Church was completed. Painted a lovely white, the wooden church had a tall bell tower that faced the mountains in many directions. To a small girl whose given name, Tomoko, meant "God Is with Me," the church steeple seemed to reach as high as the cloud-filled heavens.

2: Adventures of a Heavenly Horse

The little fish
Carried backwards,
In the clear water.
　　　　—Takai Kito

NINETEEN TWENTY-THREE was the Year of the Boar. In Japan, this year went down in history as the year of the great Kantō earthquake. Most of the industrial areas of Tokyo and Yokohama were destroyed in modern Japan's worst natural catastrophe.

Like other children born under the sign of the boar, I was very strong and fleet. Like a wild boar, I always went straight ahead toward my objective. My family and friends observed that I was good in initiating things, but when deflected I would run straight back and not always persevere. In Japan, children are given nicknames when they are two or three years old. According to my mother, when I was a baby I started to call myself Koko-chan. Today, my brothers and sisters still call me by this name.

From an early age, I loved to run, skip, dance, jump rope, and play outside. In elementary school, I always ran the first leg of the relay races, and my team usually won. As the third daughter in a family that grew to nine children, I usually managed to escape housework and generally got my way. My two older sisters, Miyako and Nobue, were expected to help Mother in the kitchen and take care of the younger children.

Once two classmates and I decided we would learn to ride a bicycle. There were no private cars or trucks in Japan at that time. Only the governor of the province had a personal automobile. In our region, there was a single truck serving five or six villages. Bicycles were just being introduced. Only men and boys rode them. Then one year a nurse in town dared to ride a bicycle to work. My girlfriends and I decided to follow her example. Father had two heavy bicycles that he used for deliveries. When they were not being used I would sneak rides without his permission. If he ever found out, he never said anything. My friends also took liberties with their fathers' or brothers' bikes. Our practices were held on the main plaza in front of the train depot. The area between the station and the elementary school was only about a hundred yards long, but it had a slight incline. While holding up each other's bikes, we mounted one at a time and let gravity do the rest. Many townspeople and schoolboys gathered to watch as we wobbled forward clutching the handlebars. When we fell off, everyone clapped.

As a result of our bold ride, we became known as the Three Tenba. In Far Eastern mythology, there is a heavenly horse known as a *tenba*. Spirited young women were often called by this name, and our appearance astride the mechanical conveyances must have seemed particularly equine. In any event, we eventually mastered the bicycle. Once we started riding, all the girls in town followed our lead.

Our family's original house was located in an old part of the village near a wooden bridge with a plaque inscribed "Castle Town." Ruins of the ancient samurai fortress looked down from a high bluff on the other side of the nearby Hi River. Up the hill near our home a path led to a small cemetery and around the corner a Buddhist temple. There was a pond near our house which was used as a reservoir in case of fire. It was very peaceful. My earliest memories are of playing near its banks, waiting for Mother in the garden nearby, or watching the sunset behind the mountains. She grew most of our vegetables, including cabbage, Chinese cabbage, scallions, string beans, albi potato, eggplant, bok choy, parsley, mustard greens, and corn. Mother was the most talkative one in the family and delighted in telling stories, keeping in touch with relatives and friends, and exchanging news with the neighbors and Members of the church. She was genuinely concerned about other people and was always selecting a fresh squash, prize *daikon*, or other produce from the garden to give to relatives and friends, teachers and doctors, and the minister and his family. In return, she would receive bamboo shoots, wild mountain grasses, and other gifts from visitors which she artfully prepared in delicious meals and snacks. She was also very active socially, serving in many capacities at church. The first one up in the morning and the last one to sleep at night, Mother always read the Bible before going to bed and kept the scriptures by her pillow. The saddest period of her life occurred when her youngest son tumbled into the pond and drowned. He was not yet three years old. I remember she wept constantly for two years until the next baby was born.

My youthful curiosity led me to explore the Hi or Chopstick River which ran through the village and was near our home. *Seri* (a red-purple plant known in the West as hemlock parsley), pussy willow, and other wild plants grew along its sandy banks. I would investigate these and follow the small streams that flowed into the river from the rice fields on either side. My love of nature and beauty often took me to the higher hills and mountain slopes in search of delicate white lilies and other wild flowers. I also looked for fiddlehead ferns, *shiitake* mushrooms, chestnuts, and other delicacies.

Once a year, in the springtime, the entire elementary school would climb the dragon mountain. It was a three- to four-hour walk each way. The peak was often shrouded in clouds and mist. It was customary to take two pairs of straw sandals for the long trek. If one pair wore out, we left them in the corner of a rice field. The old sandals, woven from rice straw, naturally returned to the soil, so the beauty of nature was not disturbed. On our backs we carried rice balls and a few pickles wrapped in bamboo skin and tied up in scarfs. In case we forgot to bring sandals along, we could easily buy something from farmhouses on the way. At the summit of the mountain, we would rest, eat our lunch, and take in the magnificent view. On a clear day, we could see the Sea of Japan. The trip back was considerably easier and lighter.

When I was about nine years old, we moved to a new, much larger house, about a half-mile away. It had formerly been an agricultural examination station. Our new home had several large rooms, a kitchen, and a bathroom as well as a small enclosed garden and abundant space outside for growing vegetables. It fronted on the main street—still a dirt road in those days—but one which carried many farmers on the way to market, schoolchildren going to class, and religious pilgrims traveling through Izumo.

Father's silkscreen factory was located behind the house in a big workshop. The farmers in Yokota and neighboring villages customarily cultivated silkworms, cotton, and linen plants and wove their own fabric. They would bring the white brocade and pick out colorful patterns that Father had designed or acquired in Kyoto. Eventually the brocade would be fashioned into kimonos, wide *obi* sashes, and other festival or holiday apparel.

Father also inscribed family crests on kimonos and made beautiful kites, flags, and pennants. The busiest time of year for our family was the period before Boys' Day, a traditional holiday that fell on May 5th. On this occasion, it was customary to unfurl flags with mythical and historic scenes and bright banners in the shape of carp. Renowned for swimming upstream, the colorful fish was a traditional symbol of ambition and perseverance—qualities admired in young males. One carp pennant would be hoisted above the house for each boy in the family. In a farming community whose bountiful annual harvest included many new children, my father's banners blew gently each spring over houses and thatched dwellings throughout the valley.

Preparation for Boys' Day began in early March. For the next two months, the whole family, including relatives and friends, helped out, from morning till evening. The flags measured about fifteen feet long by two to three feet wide, and the carp banners about three by five or six feet. We cut them from rolls of heavy cotton. Before painting, the canvas had to be pounded with a big wooden hammer over a heavy, thick, strong wooden table and then starched. When the canvas was smooth and soft, an underdesign would be composed in blue ink, usually drawn from legends, samurai stories, and scenes of famous battles. Favorite subjects included the eight-headed dragon sword, a prince from Atsuta famed for picking wild pansy, and the battle of Kawanakajima. (Lord Uesugi and Takeda, the participants in this battle, appeared as the subjects of Kurosawa's film, *Kagemusha*.). After the outline was inked in black, many different colors were used to fill in the profiles. I remember preparing sticky sweet rice starch as a base for mixing beautiful reds, greens, yellows, blues, oranges, and purples. From about age ten, I helped out, drawing the designs, and preparing the dyes. I had a keen eye and steady hand, and father soon asked me to do the first sketches. Other family members and friends would add the coloring, and father did the touching up with black ink, especially the faces.

Father also made costumes and drapes for the local theater and for pageants performed at our church. Once he made a pillow in the shape of a doll out of rice husks to collect money for the Boy Scout troop he led. Occasionally, my sister and I joined him on overnight camping expeditions to the mountains or streams. We were the only girls among a whole contingent of boys. In addition to the scout troop, Father devoted his spare time to the volunteer fire company. For many years he served as fire chief and prepared maps of the whole village.

Father was pretty successful in his work and carried a Bible whenever he took orders and made deliveries. He didn't talk much but quietly did what needed to be done. In the work-shop, I loved to help him unroll the freshly woven fabric and draw figures from myth and history. I naturally learned to make tie-dies for my dolls and draw on material. Mother also tie-dyed many of our clothes. Sometimes five or six patterns would be used on one fabric. An error could be very costly. She also tie-dyed covers for *futons*, the cotton mattresses that we slept on. From my parents, I started to develop qualities of patience and concentration that were to see me through in the years ahead.

My love of beauty and art found a rewarding outlet in this setting. Beginning in kindergarten, I had started to draw in crayon and then pencil. As a youngster, I carried a sketch book, filling up the pages with imaginative figures such as jugglers and the faces of beautiful girls. I also liked to draw vistas of rice fields and mountain forests. By high school my skill had become recognized. Boys from the neighborhood came and asked me to draw samurai faces for their kites. Still, my talent was small compared to children in Maki. Maki was a nearby village noted for its beautiful and talented children. Some of their prize-winning illustrations had been exhibited as far away as San Francisco and New York.

Religious Activities

At home I often slept in the living room by the *kotatsu*, a low-set table with a charcoal heater underneath. My futon was folded up in the morning and stored in a closet. Like most Japanese houses, there were straw *tatami* mats on the floor and an alcove known as the *tokonoma* in one side of the room for a hanging scroll of a pine tree. In the front of the living room, along the street side, my parents kept a small framed portrait of Jesus adorned in a bright red robe.

Family life centered around the church. Mr. Okazaki and Dr. Fujiwara were leaders of the whole village, not just the church, so we were always very proud. They were the richest men in the valley, and everyone respected their business acumen as well as their spiritual guidance. Even when Mr. Okazaki's bank later failed during the world-wide depression, he made sure that growing families like ours which had deposited money with him were not affected by his loss.

Our church was located about ten minutes' walk from our home, several blocks toward the center of town, past the elementary school. Its sanctuary housed a podium, an organ, a woodstove, folding chairs, and a simple wooden cross. To the side there was a stage where the choir sang and pageants were performed. In the corridor off the kitchen hung a reproduction of *L'Angelus*, a fifteenth century oil painting by François Millet showing a farmer and his wife praying in a field of ripening grain. There were also several scrolls on the walls whose firm black characters impressed resolution on our young minds. One read: "Bring Jesus to Our Village and Bring Our Village to Jesus." Another counseled: "Respecting Differences Makes for Stability." Maps of ancient Egypt and Palestine filled the opposite wall. In church school we memorized places mentioned in the scriptures and played a card game with pictures of Moses, Joseph, Samuel, Ruth and Naomi, and other Biblical characters to help us prepare for weekly tests. I especially loved the songs of David. Growing up, I felt the Holy Land close to my heart. I imagined that its valleys of plenty were like my own homeland of Izumo.

On Thursday evenings we assembled at church for choir practice and throughout the year met there for other celebrations. The most important was Christmas when the congregation assembled for a Nativity pageant reenacting Joseph and Mary's quest for shelter at the inn, the birth of the baby Jesus in a manger, and the arrival of the three wise men from the East. We all sang Christmas carols on the stage around a large Christmas tree gaily decorated with small dolls and other ornaments. The church gave us presents. In the fifth grade, I received a big Bible, which I used all the time until its binding tore. For Christmas dinner, Mother always made *gomoku meshi*, a rice casserole with carrots, burdock, and small delicate shellfish that came from Lake Shinjiko in Matsue.

How I looked forward to Christmas with Miyako and Nobue and my younger brothers and sisters, Makoto, Atsumi, Junko, Kyū, Masaru, and Yoko. With the exception of holi-

days, our greatest thrill was climbing up the church bell
tower. The stairs were high and narrow, and to a small girl
or boy it seemed like ascending the ladder to heaven. The bell
had a beautiful sound. In addition to regular services it was
rung at Christmas and Easter.

The timeless cycle of planting and harvest governed life in
our village as throughout the Far East. Although our family
was Christian, we celebrated other traditional religious festivals and holidays, seeing all faiths as expressions of one
universal spirit. Most of the Shintō festivals fell at harvest
time, but one took place in the spring. Several miles east of
the village there was an old shrine known as Tenjinsan, built
a thousand years ago. It was dedicated to Michizane Sugahara,
a loyal Imperial minister who was exiled to Kyushu, Japan's
southernmost island, after losing a famous battle. Tenjinsan's
festival was held in the early spring when the plum trees
blossomed. I especially loved the Shintō dances based on songs
from the *Kojiki* and other ancient texts. Years later, I recognized some similarity between the Japanese dances and
Nepalese and Kashmiri folk dances in the Himalayas. Food
was plentiful and delicious at these autumnal festivals. With
my brothers and sisters I would stock up on mochi, fried tofu,
nishime-style wild grasses, forest mushrooms, and other plants
that were foraged at this time. Sake also flowed freely. But
of course as Salvationists, we did not partake of anything
stronger than tea.

When I was in the fourth grade, a new shrine to Princess
Kushi-Inada-Hime was built on the outskirts of town. I used
to ride my bicycle past the rice fields to the site, about two
miles away. Its approach was lined with gorgeous cherry
trees and flanked by a high *torii* gate, wind towers, and
a stone lantern. People traditionally came to the large wooden
shrine with its long sloping roof in hope of safe childbirth.
Sacred bamboo from a nearby pond was traditionally sent to
the Imperial Palace in Kyoto and later Tokyo to ease the
deliveries of the Empress or her daughters. During festivals
reenacting the tales from the *Kojiki*, about twenty people would

dress up in a gigantic dragon costume and parade from the village to the shrine. I vividly remember the ceremony at the shrine of Princess Kushi-Inada-Hime, especially the beautiful and peaceful *kagura* dance.

Holidays and Festivals

Elsewhere in the valley was a twelve-hundred-year-old Esoteric Buddhist temple built by Kūkai, a famous priest from Koyasan. It was one of the oldest Shingon temples in Japan, and in the stone was a footstep that was said to have been made when Kūkai fell to earth from heaven. There was also a Buddhist temple that had been most recently rebuilt about one hundred and fifty years ago. It had a lofty ginkgo tree in its courtyard. On New Year's Eve, the temple bell would ring one hundred and eight times to help purify the valley of delusions. Its deep reverberations could be heard for miles around. On New Year's Eve, we stayed up late like families across Japan to welcome the New Year in with bowls of hot homemade *soba* noodles and broth.

In the countryside where wealth was measured by the annual harvest, the local economy functioned principally on credit. Twice a year, at the Bon Festival on July 15 and at the end of the lunar calendar in December, credit vouchers were tallied up and exchanged for cash. Like the other children in the family, I was expected to help out with collections but always found it embarrassing to ask for money. Meanwhile, at home, our parents' bills also came due. There was always great relief when the rice bill, the family's biggest expense, was met.

The rice came in big cotton sacks, and we ate it at almost every meal along with miso soup, cooked vegetables from land and sea, and raw pickles. It was very good quality rice, only lightly milled, and of course grown without any chemical fertilizers or artificial pesticides. Mother cooked rice in the traditional manner, in a big cast-iron pot suspended from the ceiling over a wood fire that was gradually replaced with charcoal to provide a low, even heat. A heavy wooden lid weighing ten to twenty pounds was put over the rice pot, and often a large stone, to provide pressure. In preparation for the New Year, we helped Mother make mochi. For days beforehand, we pounded hundreds of pounds of steamed sweet rice with a heavy wooden pestle. The mochi would be enjoyed throughout the month of January, with strips of *nori* seaweed, a little bonito fish flakes, a touch of grated daikon mixed with tamari soy sauce, or chopped scallions. At this time, we also enjoyed sweet azuki beans, tarts made with *kinako*, or roasted soy flour, and chestnuts.

On New Year's Day, after visiting a local shrine, we gathered with relatives and friends for feasting, games, and merriment. We enjoyed playing *Hyakunin Isshu*, a traditional New Year's card game in which the two sides competed to match and recite lines and verses from one hundred famous poems. Even today, I can still recall by heart about fifty to sixty of the poems drawn from anthologies such as the *Manyōshu*, the *Kokinshu*, and the poems of Kakinomoto Hitomaro and Lady Murasaki. This game was one of the few times during which boys and girls played together. Among the older children, teenagers, and parents, there was much matchmaking going on. The card game included many tender love poems. Matching these with the opposite sex assumed an aura of excitement and romance.

The next major holiday, Girls' Day, fell in the spring, on March 3. On this occasion, dolls were set out in each household representing the Emperor, Empress, five musicians and five warriors. The chief recreation, *Hagoita*, or Japanese badminton, was played outdoors with light, square wooden racquets. Mine had the picture of a beautiful lady on the back. The shuttlecock was made of a big black seed and feathers. Attired in long-sleeved kimonos, the girls and young ladies were very beautiful to watch playing this graceful game, and we received many compliments. Refreshments consisted of homemade *amazaké*, mugwort mochi, and savory spring grasses.

On Buddha's birthday, April 8, children customarily went to the temple to receive a gift of *amacha*, a delicious beverage made from sweet tea leaves. With the other boys and girls, we also poured *amacha* tea over the big Sakyamuni Buddha statue. It was said to have healing properties.

In midsummer, beginning July 15, Japanese traditionally observed a week in honor of their ancestors. At the cemetery, big bonfires were made to welcome back the souls of the departed. At home, an altar would be erected containing the loved one's picture and cherished personal effects. Incense would be lit and many beautiful lanterns—some long, others round—would be strung up, adding a fragrant aroma and radiant glow to the occasion. As Christians, our home didn't contain the ordinary Shintō and Buddhist altars found in most households. But at this time of year we prepared a special altar in the alcove in the front room. It was customary to make *bon-dango*, partially kneaded sweet rice flour, steamed, and rolled in yellow soy flour. Several *dango* would be skewered like shish kebab and put in front of the altar or by the burial site for the returning spirits. From an early age, we grew up with the understanding of food as spiritual energy as well as physical nourishment.

At the end of the solar calendar in July, there was a big sporting event in Yokota known as Inyo (Yin-Yang) Tennis Tournament. People came from throughout the valley to watch. It was sponsored in part by Mr. Okazaki, who was influenced by Western art and culture besides religion and medicine. Though it was rare for women to play tennis at that time, there was a very strong woman player, Mitsuko Yodono. Mitsuko, a relative of Mr. Okazaki, was about ten years older than me. As a child I admired her very much. On and off the playing field, she was a true *tenba*, or heavenly horse. I never dreamed that in the years ahead she was to play a pivotal role in my future development.

One of Mr. Okazaki's sons later became an excellent tennis player. Known as Ken-chan, he had been born a few weeks after me. We grew up practically as brother and sister. His brother was a beautiful singer and led the chorus in church. Growing up, Ken-chan was always very active and exuberant. Mr. Hata, my fifth and sixth grade elementary school teacher, was also very active on the tennis courts. He had both a strong serve and volley. Father enjoyed watching tennis with us children, but his big love was *sumo*, or Japanese-style wrestling. It was very popular, and boys competed in a tournament from the fourth grade on. Most of the boys and young men were of ordinary size and weight, not tremendously fat like the famous sumo wrestlers today. Wrestling tournaments were popular attractions during festivals at shrines.

At the end of November there was a big agricultural festival in town that drew farmers from all around to exchange new-born calves. The Cow Market was held in a large green field between the school and hospital. Hundreds of people came, and temporary market stalls sprouted along the street featuring ceramics, kimonos, and food of all kinds. Of course, in those days, cattle were used exclusively for farming, as an energy source. Beef and dairy food were not traditionally consumed in Japan or the Orient. Only one farmer in the valley kept a dairy cow. He supplied milk to a handful of those who had been influenced by modern civilization and wanted to try it for pleasure or for medicinal purposes. In our family, we had meat—usually rabbit or wild game—about once or twice a year. Poultry and eggs were also very rare. We had fish and seafood more frequently. Yokota was considerably inland. In the days before refrigeration and rapid transport, food from the sea was a special treat.

For the first ten years, my life was confined to the beautiful mountain valley where I was born and grew up. In the sixth grade, I accompanied my classmates on an outing to Matsue, the capital of Izumo province. For the first time I visited a modern city, saw endless numbers of houses and people, passed stores with the latest Western fashions, and caught a glimpse of a wider, but divided world.

3: Lessons of a Peasant Sage

"If you work hard and faithfully at this great task
[rice cultivation], you will be free from hunger and
starvation from generation to generation. Do not
ask for any short cut. In the final analysis Heaven
has its own natural way of doing things, and in order
to obtain rice the only proper procedure is to culti-
vate rice plants."—Sontoku Ninomiya

THERE WAS a Far Eastern saying: "When seeking a
teacher, do not mind traveling a thousand miles." As
a student, it was my favorite proverb.

From age six to eleven, I studied at the local grammar
school in Yokota and then attended high school from age
twelve to thirteen. The Japanese language is easy to speak
but difficult to write. In school, we spent a lot of time copy-
ing, memorizing, and chanting the different characters and
ideograms. These included two sets of *kana*, made up of forty-
six phonetic characters each, and several thousand *kanji*,
Chinese ideograms. There were about thirty children altogether
in my class. Until the third grade, boys and girls studied
together. From the fourth through sixth grades, they were
divided. The number of students in high school, both boys and
girls, fell sharply as many young people left to help out in
the fields.

In a rural community, it was especially rare for a girl to
go to college in those days. Generally only the wealthy
could afford higher education. I didn't know whether my
parents could pay for my tuition and expenses, but I really
wanted to go. With two other girls, I studied after class my

last year in high school to prepare for the college examinations. The other girls were a year older than me and had taken a year off after graduating from high school to study for the exams. The written tests covered proficiency in Japanese language, history, and mathematics. To my surprise, I not only passed the examination but received the highest marks of seventy applicants that year. My study partner, Keiko Tamura, came in second. Her mother was a teacher, and she was very smart. The other girl, Tamiko Onda, also passed. She was the daughter of a Shintō priest.

Although college was expensive and there were many children to support, Father decided to send me. Mother was against the idea and wanted me to stay and get a job. But I was determined to see a wider world and saw teaching as a noble career.

I received a small scholarship, lightening the burden somewhat on my parents. In April 1938, I left for the Women's Teachers' College in Hamada. A large coastal city on the Sea of Japan, Hamada was a five-hour journey through the mountains by train. My family and friends saw me off at the platform, and we waved to each other until the old black steam-driven locomotive chugged out of sight.

By any standards, Hamada was a big city. For a country girl like me, its broad avenues, bustling stores and restaurants, and large army base were a constant source of new impressions. It was also located on the coast in the direction of the Izumo Shrine. I had visited the shrine once in my youth. Dedicated to the offspring of Princess Kushi-Inada-Hime and Susa-no-wo, it was the oldest shrine in Japan. Because of their marriage, it was a favorite pilgrimage site for honeymoons and weddings. The month of October we call *kannazuki*, meaning "month without god." From all over Japan, gods and goddesses including Amaterasu, the Sun Goddess came to Izumo to meet. For centuries, people came to this quiet and peaceful site for her blessing.

The college was located about half a mile inland from the waterfront. The dormitory, a large two-story building adjacent to the classrooms, was to be my home for the next six years. There were two systems of teacher training. The first, in which I was enrolled, consisted of five years of study, followed by a year of graduate work. The second was a two-year graduate program for those who had attended a junior college elsewhere. My class consisted of about thirty girls. Seven of us shared a single small room in the dormitory, and during the day our futons were folded up and stored in a closet. Altogether about one hundred fifty girls were enrolled at the school. Next to the campus there was an elementary school for practice teaching. The Men's Teachers' College was located in Matsue, the capital of Izumo province, about one hundred miles along the coastline further east. There was virtually no contact between students at the two schools.

Classes met five times a day, six days a week. The curriculum, designed on the German and French model, was rigorous and included Japanese, Chinese, English, science, history (Far Eastern and Western), geography, philosophy, mathematics, home economics, art, music, and gymnastics. In the third year, we also studied philosophy and education. The principal, class adviser, and most of our teachers were gentlemen. There were a few lady instructors, who taught primarily cooking, sewing, music, and English.

In the 1890s, the Meiji Emperor had issued a Rescript on Education that the headmaster and students of each school were expected to chant every morning: "The Way here set forth is indeed the teaching bequeathed by Our Imperial Ancestors, to be observed alike by Their Descendants and the subjects, infallible for all ages and true in all places."

One of the most important courses, *Shūshin*, or ethics, emphasized spiritual values and attitudes. It consisted of moral instruction, proverbs, and lessons drawn from the lives of saints, heroes, and famous people. Across Japan, students from grammar school through college were expected to attend Shūshin twice a week and develop their character. In college, we kept diaries in which we evaluated our daily thoughts and behavior. A white circle meant a bright day, a black circle

a bad day, and a half black/half white circle a partly sunny/
partly cloudy day.

Usually the school's principal or senior teachers would
conduct Shūshin, emphasizing obedience to parents, respect
for ancestors, and loyalty to the nation. In addition to stories
about great samurai and shōguns and patriotic generals and
admirals, we studied the maxims of ancient sages like Lao
Tzu and Confucius, as well as modern reformers such as
Sontoku Ninomiya and Sagen Ishizuka. Exemplary Western
thinkers and leaders were also presented from time to time,
including Gutenberg, Isaac Newton, Benjamin Franklin, and
Abraham Lincoln. From an early age, the story of how George
Washington told the truth to his father about cutting down
the cherry blossoms made a deep impression. I came to see
America not just as the land of cowboys and Indians, baseball
and Hollywood movies. It was also home for statesmen of
filial devotion and moral vision.

College Studies

History was my favorite subject. We studied Chinese history
the first year, Western history the second year, and Japanese
history the third year. We also studied the Far Eastern classics. I especially liked the Japanese classics and avidly studied
many books and poems. My favorite poems, by Hitomaro
Kakinomoto, came from the *Manyōshu*, an anthology composed in the Hamada area some twelve hundred years earlier.
A Buddhist monk, who lived about six hundred years before
my time, also wrote beautifully and attracted me very much.
From the third year, the teachers didn't allow us to use a
dictionary. Since classical Japanese differed from the modern
language, it was difficult in the beginning, rather like reading
Geoffrey Chaucer in the West. But after writing out selections
from the old texts and reading them a hundred times, we
began to understand. Often I composed my own verses and
put them together in little handmade books of poetry.

We also read translations of Western novels, including

works by Tolstoy, Dostoevsky, and Dickens. I particularly liked *Uncle Tom's Cabin* by Harriet Beecher Stowe. Her moral fervor and social responsibility reminded me of the Salvation Army. I also enjoyed Pearl Buck's *The Good Earth*.

One of our favorite Western authors, Lafcadio Hearn, was a local legend and sage. At the end of the nineteenth century, Hearn came to Japan from America and settled in Matsue where he began to write about the legends and lore of old Japan. His folk tales, ghost stories, and other romances centered around Izumo, which he described as "the ancient province of the gods." Adopting the Japanese name Yakumo, which means "Eight Clouds or Overlapping Clouds," he married a Japanese woman and had a family. He spent the rest of his life trying to preserve the memory of old Japan. Between the intellect of the modern and traditional mind, he observed, "there is a psychological interval as hopeless as the distance from planet to planet."

Hearn's tiny writing studio across from the old castle in Matsue has been preserved as a museum. After his death, he was given a posthumous name meaning "Believing Man Similar to the Undefiled Flower Blooming like Eight Rising Clouds who Dwells in the Mansion of Right Enlightenment." Hearn's love of nature and devotion to the harmonious meeting of East and West were a beacon for several generations of Japanese schoolchildren in addition to American readers. I particularly liked his description of the pounding of the big rice pestles for which Izumo was famous. "It is the beating of the pulse of the land," he wrote, "like a heart beat in its regularity." Hearn's niece, Koizumi, was in our school, and from her we learned firsthand about this unusual man.

Though I excelled in literature, I got off to a rather inauspicious start in art. In my first class, I sketched a ceramic pot, and my teacher became angry. It turned out to be a Korean pot. Located directly across from Izumo on the other side of the Sea of Japan, Korea at that time was a colony of Japan, and feelings against everything Korean ran strong. Moreover, the pot was the kind used as a urinal.

In calligraphy, I initially didn't fare much better. My instructor laughed at my efforts. But in my third year of classes, a wonderful calligraphy teacher arrived and nurtured my development. I became keenly devoted to the writing brush and ink, and in the grammar school next door learned my ABC's along with the young pupils. Once, on vacation, at home in Yokota, I practiced a thousand characters a day. My new love of calligraphy and rapid development taught me the value of teaching. Children really change as a result of their teacher's inspiration.

I wasn't so good in the exact sciences. I didn't care for math or chemistry at all. Biology was more interesting, and I enjoyed going on field excursions in search of wild grasses.

Music was also an important part of the curriculum. There was an organ at school to teach the children to sing. Pianos were very expensive. On this organ we practiced "do, re, me, fa, sol, . . ." and other scales as well as classical music, folk songs, and ballads. We learned simple arrangements by Bach, Beethoven, Mozart, and Haydn. I especially liked Russian folk songs, besides those from England, Scotland, Ireland, France, and Italy. Years later when I went to Germany for the first time, I was very impressed with the natural environment. I could hear "Lorelei" and the other tunes I studied years before arising from the land, the rivers, and the mountains.

We didn't study traditional Japanese songs and dances. Compared to Western music, they were very complex. But we studied Noh drama as literature. It wasn't until twenty-five years later in the United States that I really came to appreciate this traditional aspect of Japan.

Among American folk songs, I delighted in Stephen C. Foster's ballads such as "Oh, Suzanna." Even though we sang the words in Japanese, the rhythm and melody had a lyrical quality that made them enjoyable in any language. We also studied dance, including ballet and modern styles.

American movies came to Hamada at this time, and as often as possible we would go to the local cinema in town. We saw *Gone with the Wind, Casablanca,* and *The Girl in the Orchestra* and at school parties dressed up and imitated the mannerisms of Maureen O'Hara, Clark Gable, Humphrey Bogart, Ingrid Bergman, Deanna Durban, and other giants of the silver screen. Some girls were so infatuated that after the college gates closed at 5 P.M. they would climb the wooden fence and sneak off to the movies downtown, returning just before late-night inspection and lights out at 10 P.M. Sometimes they would line up still wearing silk stockings they had put on for their outings. The teacher wisely let their fancy attire pass unobserved.

Once a year in the dorm, we had a big festival. Each class gave a skit on stage. As chairman of my class for five years, I also served as director, organizing the dramas, scenery, and costumes. The first year, we did a scene from *Casablanca*. The second year, we performed a scene from a Bette Davis film. The third year, we drew upon *A Doll's House* by Ibsen, who was my favorite playwright. The fourth year, I became enthralled with a play entitled *The Priest and His Disciple* about Shinran, a famous Buddhist monk and the first shōgun of the Kamakura era. The first time I read it, I couldn't put it down. After everyone else went to sleep at ten o'clock, I continued to read it in a closet with a flashlight the whole night, tears streaming down my cheeks. I loved it so much I wanted to produce it for the class skit. But it was very serious, and most of the other girls wanted something more fun. My choice prevailed, and the faculty congratulated us for our perform-ance.

The fifth year I created my own play, coinciding with the 2600-year anniversary celebration of Japan. It included scenes from mythology and history up to modern times. From the *Kojiki* I selected the tale of how Amaterasu, the Sun Goddess, became very angry when her brothers killed some animals and hid in a cave. Worried that Japan had become so dark, the rest of the gods made a fire and danced, luring her out of the cave with the sacred mirror in which she saw her own reflection. I choreographed the dance with the beating of a drum, and for the first time I myself performed on stage.

48

Ninomiya's Teachings

At the end of the third year, the principal changed. The
first had been very gentle and skinny, a typical old gentleman
of the Taishō (1912–1926) era. The new principal, Mr.
Watanabe, was strong and active. With him he brought
Moichi Tanaka, a new education teacher, who became our
class adviser and the major influence on my overall college
education and development.

Mr. Tanaka was twenty-nine when he arrived at our campus
fresh from Senior Teachers' College. He was originally from
Hagi City, a place many educators came out of during the
turbulent events leading up to the Meiji era. One of them,
Shōin Yoshida, had been martyred at age thirty by the last
shōgun for calling for an end to feudalism and relations with
the West. Statues commemorating Yoshida's selfless spirit
were erected in elementary and high schools across Japan following the Meiji Restoration. We grew up inspired by his
vision of Japan as part of a harmonious international order.

But it was another reformer, Sontoku Ninomiya, who was
to be the major influence on Mr. Tanaka, our principal
Mr. Watanabe, and our class. Born in 1787, Ninomiya grew
up within sight of Mt. Fuji and remained a farmer his whole
life. Blessed with native common sense and deep intuition, he
taught that agricultural labor is the noblest of human en-
deavors, and that for it to succeed farmers must cooperate
unselfishly and share their harvest and resources. Until his
death in 1856, Ninomiya worked tirelessly. He established
rural cooperatives, which he called Societies for the Repay-
ment of Virtue, and saved many rural communities from
starvation and economic ruin. Ninomiya's devotion to nature
and practical approach to the problems of society inspired
future generations. Communes based on his ideals spread
across the country and earned him the name "Peasant Sage
of Japan."

Still, eighty years after his death, Ninomiya's teaching,
known as *Hōtoku*, or "Returning Gratitude," was very strong.
Like the Bible, my copy of his book was so well read that it

was worn down. I still have it. The study of his teachings changed our lives. In the first and second year of college, we studied Kant, Hegel, and other Western philosophers, but I couldn't catch their teachings very well. Then we studied Ninomiya, and his words were simple and direct. His observations sprang from a deep understanding of the natural order and served as wonderful reflections for daily life. I still remember by heart many of his poems:

Rice and cotton clothing and miso soup are helping you.
More than that is destroying you.

*

If you hear mice crying,
You understand that for mice that is hell.
For cats, it is paradise.

*

People try to study Buddhist sutras, the Tao
    Teh Ching, and I Ching by reading.
But real life is not in books.
One must see nature itself. That is the best book.

In our fourth and fifth years, our education was based on Ninomiya's teachings, and our dorm operated on Hōtoku principles. Instead of criticizing, Ninomiya taught that you should emphasize the positive. At our dorm meetings, we would talk only about our classmates' and teachers' good points. Ninomiya encouraged spontaneity and initiative rather than duties and obligations. In the dorm, we began to clean and take responsibility for common areas and perform personal tasks without schedules or reminders. Ninomiya observed that a wise teacher or leader watched over and guided others but did not tell them what to do. In class, the soft-spoken Mr. Tanaka would allow us to create and learn for ourselves, rather than drill us in a particular subject. He would propose topics for study but let us select and discuss them ourselves. Only afterward would he give his own comment.

As chairman of my dorm, I also tried to adopt this method

even though it ran counter to my wild boar nature. For example, we used to individually take out the sewage and put it in the garden. After meeting together, we came up with a much better method. The Education Department heard about the changes we were making. They were written up in an educational periodical and brought positive responses from all over Japan.

In Hamada there was no Salvation Army Church, so I didn't attend religious services regularly. I visited other Protestant and Catholic services on occasion but became more interested in Japanese classics. On Sunday afternoons, Mr. Tanaka held open house at his private residence, and his wife served refreshments. One New Year's, visiting his home with seven classmates, I drank sake for the first time.

Sports and Outings

Sports took up the rest of our free moments. There were four clubs for students: tennis, volleyball, basketball, and swimming. Yokota was famous for a big tennis tournament that took place every year at the end of July. The whole region came to watch it. In college, I naturally joined the tennis club and by the third year started competing with teams from other colleges.

But my real love was gymnastics. Other colleges had gym classes or clubs, but for some reason ours did not. As the war progressed, we could not buy tennis balls or racquets. I began to organize a gymnastics club. We didn't need anything new. The school already had equipment. I recruited and trained the girls myself. We exercised to music and carried out callisthenics and exercises on the jumping horse, parallel bars, and balance beam. I particularly liked the balance beam, which was made of wood. I would mount its high bar, turn around, ending up with a hand stand. We also studied the martial arts, including lady's long sword and archery, volleyball, and track and field.

In the foreword to a small poetry book I compiled many

years later, Mr. Tanaka recalled of this period:

> Miss Yokoyama's passion was concentrated into gym-
> nastics. She called upon the other students and established
> the Gymnastics Club at school. Many of her schoolmates
> in the same class and lower-class students acted in co-
> operation with her proposal. They eagerly practiced
> every day until dark as if they were possessed. It looked
> like a strong religious group, which could be called the
> "Yokoyama Sect" rather than a simple gymnastics club.
> This was all created through her ability and character.
> She was active by nature and broad-minded, enjoying the
> confidence of students for her warm heart and never
> speaking ill of other people.

One of the regular athletic instructors, Mr. Shiraiwa, who
had recently joined the faculty, eventually instructed us and
became our club's adviser. He emphasized sports as a spiritual
discipline unifying mind and body. When he first saw me, he
observed that I was too short, too fat, and my legs were too
big to be much of an athlete. But my running, jumping (for
both height and distance), and tennis amazed him. In 1941,
our gymnastics team became champions, and in November,
just a month before Pearl Harbor, we went to Tokyo for the
National Olympics. It was a great honor to be selected, but
we were no match for a Japanese girls' gymnastics squad from
Manchuria. They had Chinese or Russian instructors and were
the number one team in their region. They were so beautiful
to look at, we just watched.

Forty years later, on a visit to Japan, I looked up my
gymnastics teacher. He recalled "the laughing sound" of my
"clear, beautiful voice" and remembered me as "a really
special athlete, good student, and leader whom everyone
followed." In college, I began to notice that my inner drive
as well as small physical size was different from my classmates.
Part of my leadership abilities came from my birth year. The
Japanese school year begins in April, while the Oriental as-

trology calendar begins in February. Since I was born at the
end of February, I grew up with classmates almost a year
older than myself. They were almost all born in the Year of
the Dog and were happy to follow the lead of someone with
the determination of a wild boar.

Trips and outings provided another outlet for my organizing skills and opportunity to indulge my love of the outdoors.
During the regular term, our favorite getaway spot was Dove
Tail Hill on the waterfront about fifteen minutes' walk from
campus. We used to swim in the harbor, with its old fishing
boats, tangled seaweed, and soaring ospreys. There was a
small Shintō shrine on the hill, and a gnarled pine tree that
jutted out over the bluff. The bright yellow dandelions, purple
azaleas, and other flowers on the shoreline, along with the
lapping of the water and salty breeze, made this a special spot
to relax, study, or sketch.

Our first principal, the elderly gentleman, recommended
daily constitutionals. Once, with him at our head, we all
walked from Hamada to Gotsu, the next big town, about
forty miles along the coast. Our destination was a Shintō
shrine, and we walked all morning and afternoon. After paying
our respects we came back by train the same night. On another
occasion, we visited a movie studio and recognized a famous
actress at the railroad station. In their excitement, some of
my classmates followed the film star, and our adviser became
incensed.

Another time our class went to Yoshino at cherry blossom
time in early May. The gymnastics teacher and I organized
the expedition. One morning at 4 A.M. we led four com-
panions up a deep mountainside to visit the eight-hundred-
year-old dwelling of a famous Buddhist monk.

Actually this trip was part of our annual class tour. At the
conclusion of the spring term, every class would organize
a journey to some memorable cultural and historical part of
the country. From Yoshino we went to Tokyo to visit the
dōjō, or training center, of the gymnastics teacher. Mr.
Watanabe, the new principal, met us there and told us how

much he liked our class. He said our devotion to Ninomiya's ideals and the friendship we shared with one another were unique. However, by the end of the two-week trip we were all so tired that we didn't even want to take pictures when we reached the last major stop, Kyoto.

The next year we planned to visit Kyushu, Japan's southernmost island. But Kyushu was a staging area for military operations in China, and our trip was cancelled. Instead, we decided to visit Tokyo again and see government leaders. Our adviser reminded us that there was a big war in Asia underway and busy ministers had no time for country girls. But I pushed for it. With five or six friends, I stayed up late one night after lights out to write letters to the cabinet officials. To our delight, they replied, "Please come, we are waiting to welcome you." Our teacher was amazed and said we were really an unusual class.

In preparation for our visit, the teacher taught us table manners and other proprieties that were practiced in the nation's capital. He showed us how to eat an apple correctly and how to slice a banana. He told us to cut one piece at a time, lay the knife down, and swallow it before cutting the next slice. At the National Diet in Tokyo we were greeted cordially by the Prime Minister and other top ministers. They invited us to come to a big banquet. There we sat down while waiters, dressed in black ties and shirts, stood behind us serving Western-style courses. Our trip was a huge success, and we were brimming with pride.

At the time of our visit to Tokyo, in spring 1940, the war with China had grown intense. Relations with the United States, Britain, and France were deteriorating. Until this time, right up to the end of the 1930s, things had been pretty free and liberal, at least in Izumo province, even though we faced toward Korea and the Manchurian coast. During the first two years of college, there was not much nationalist influence, but in the third year military preparations began.

Hamada was home to a big army base, number 21. Marches and drills were held frequently, and an atmosphere of discipline began to prevail. Our class increasingly went as a unit to the railroad station with a flag to see off soldiers bound for the frontlines in China and Manchuria. One day there was a memorial procession to the grave of a young soldier who had died, and one of my classmates decided to fast.

Still, the war was a long way away, the stuff of newspaper headlines and radio bulletins. We had no notion of the long years of loss and sacrifice ahead. Pearl Harbor came as a complete shock, to the Japanese no less than the Americans. I remember running frantically through the dorm spreading the news to others as soon as I heard it. With the entry of the United States into the war, everything changed. Suddenly, everyone wore long faces. Rationing of rice, soy sauce, salt, charcoal, matches, and other basics began. We no longer were allowed to receive individual food parcels from our families. The tennis courts at school were dug up and turned into gardens to grow Chinese cabbage, sweet potatoes, and other food.

Overnight everything American became decadent and alien. Movies ceased. Western-style beauty parlors that turned straight Japanese hair into cascades of curls closed. Even the American-style mop and wax we used to clean the floors were thrown out in favor of old-fashioned napkins and elbow-grease. At school our English teacher was accused of promoting enemy styles of fashion. She had her hair in a permanent and wore red dresses and high heels. She was the one whose clothes we borrowed to dress up as movie stars. We all felt sorry for her. But we were happy when English classes were cancelled. English was our most difficult subject.

As the war in the Pacific got under way, we would go barefoot at 6 A.M. each day, even in winter, to the nearby shrine to worship and express our gratitude to the soldiers who had died in battle. For the next two years, we joined with the soldiers in daily drilling. We wore *mompe*, the baggy trousers that became the uniform of women in Japan during the rest of the war.

The austerity of wartime entertainment was partially relieved by exciting stories of Miyamoto Musashi, Japan's most famous samurai, whose exploits were serialized every morning in the daily newspaper. The great sword master had a young boy who tagged along after him named Jōtaro. My classmates nicknamed me Jōtaro and rushed downstairs every morning to read the latest installment and compare my tomboyish ways with his adventures.

Despite official optimism and news of ever bigger victories for the Japanese Imperial Forces, there were signs of defeat. Mr. Tanaka confided to us that the army was really degenerating within and could not protect the country for very long. As we graduated to an uncertain future, he told us that the destiny of Japan—and the world—would be determined by the next generation of educators whose ranks we had just entered.

4: Memories of Clouds Passing By

"The bell of the Gion Temple tolls into every man's
heart to warn him that all is vanity and evanescence.
The faded flowers of the sala trees by the Buddha's
death-bed bear witness to the truth that all who
flourish are destined to decay. Yes, pride must have
its fall, for it is as unsubstantial as a dream on a
spring night. The brave and violent man—he too
must die away in the end, like a whirl of dust in
the wind." —*The Tale of the Heike*

AFTER COMPLETING graduate school, I left Hamada and
returned home to teach. For Japan, the war in the Pacific
had taken a turn for the worse. American forces had
captured Saipan, and land-based B-29s were now in striking
range of the country. Though Izumo remained untouched by
the bombing, daily life grew more austere, and family and
friends became caught up in the war effort.

While I was still in college, Miyako, my eldest sister, left
home to attend designers' school. She had a talent for dressmaking and stayed with an aunt in Yonago, a coastal city
located near Matsue. Before completing her studies, she
departed for a Salvation Army training school and married a
Salvation Army officer. During the war, he was sent to
Manchuria to aid the Japanese army in a civilian capacity.
Miyako accompanied him to Dairen, a port in Manchuria,
where they had two sons.

My next eldest sister, Nobue, remained for a while in
Yokota, working for a railroad express company near the

station. As a girl she had always been very strong and active, running the last lap of the relay races with me at elementary school. The boys in class were actually afraid of her, and when she came to warm her hands by a bonfire in the schoolyard they would slip away. With so many men and boys called into the armed forces, manual labor was scarce. Her job involved a lot of heavy lifting, but she was up to the task. Through relatives, a marriage was arranged for Nobue with a guard stationed on the Manchurian-Siberian border. She left to join him. Though brave at heart, she wept on leaving. Friends accompanying her reported that tears streamed down her cheeks as the boat left to cross the Sea of Japan.

My younger brother, Makoto, enlisted in the Naval Air Corps and was dispatched to China. Brought up under the watchful eye of three older sisters, he had reserves of patience and endurance. My younger sister, Junko, followed my footsteps and enrolled in Teachers' College in Hamada. But as the war progressed, she was drafted and assigned to work at an aircraft manufacturing plant in Nagoya. The other children were too small to be directly affected by the mobilization and stayed at home.

Father and Mother also remained in Yokota, devoting more and more time to religious activities. Our church had been particularly hard hit by the war. The government had requisitioned the gongs, bells, and altarpieces of all shrines and temples in the country. The beautiful big bell in our church tower was melted down and recast into weaponry. The minister had left or been drafted, and national feeling turned against Christianity, which was seen as the religion of the enemy. During the war, all Protestant congregations united, and services were often held in private. One of Mr. Okazaki's sons served as temporary minister.

Mitsuko Yodono, the young tennis star whom I admired as a child, went off to Brazil with her husband after graduating from a foreign language college in Yokohama. When the war broke out, they came back and volunteered for duty in Manchuria. Like many Japanese stationed abroad at this time, their family, which included several small children, accompanied them. Several of my classmates from Teachers' College also left for the Asian mainland to serve as instructors for Japanese dependents or to accompany their husbands.

My first teaching assignment was a class of ten- and eleven-year-old girls at the elementary school in Maki, an isolated mountain village about ten miles from Yokota. Since olden days, Maki had been known for its beautiful women. After the famous battle of Gen-Pei, some of the defeated survivors of the Heike clan hid among the villagers. The story of those times is told in the *Heike monogatari* (The Tale of the Heike), one of the classics of Japanese literature. The epic's opening verse, describing the tolling of a Buddhist temple bell in India, has been recited for nine hundred years.

Whether or not they were descended from the former rulers of the imperial court in Kyoto, the girls I taught came from surrounding farms and had a cheerful, meek nature. Growing up on grains and vegetables, spring water, and occasional trout from the mountain streams, they were healthy and energetic. In addition to the regular curriculum, they performed skits and went on field trips and overnight expeditions to collect wild plants with their new teacher. In cleaning up, taking out sewage, and other common tasks at school, I tried to instill principles of trust and cooperation, besides impressing on them the dignity of labor I had learned from Ninomiya's teachings.

As the call-up of men and boys continued, the children were needed to help with the planting and harvest. Many times the whole class went to the rice fields to help farmers. In the springtime, we would cut brush for fertilizer and then press it down in the mud with our feet. Working outdoors together made us very happy. In the fields, the children's eyes shone brightly in wonder and satisfaction. Back in the classroom, I encouraged the girls to make sketches of daily life. Supplies were very scarce during the war. We didn't have normal drawing paper and made do with straw-backed paper that could easily be broken. The children went about their illustrations quietly, while I looked over their work from time to time. I saved their pictures for several years. But today only one survives—a small drawing of a traditional charcoal fire.

During lunch, I checked my pupils' diaries and copied some of their poems on the blackboard. I had always enjoyed *haiku* and the longer 31-syllable *waka* and encouraged them to express their thoughts in verse. After lunch, we would read and discuss the poems together. The children's haiku were so beautiful and natural that I copied them down in my own notebook at night. They were much better than adults' poems. I could feel the children's pure, naive souls. Their minds were more beautiful than the mountain and clearer than the river. In later years, I showed them to some teachers at a haiku society who agreed they were exceptional.

Maki was located on the roof of the Chūgoku mountains on the border of Hiroshima Prefecture. There were several ways to enter the village. The mountain pass that I took when I commuted from Yokota was big and crooked. The long dirt road curved around seven or eight hills leading up from the valley. Just beyond the peak of the pass, beautiful Maki Basin appeared below. Pushing my father's heavy bicycle, I would go up the pass, wiping the perspiration from my face. It was tiring, but the joyful thought of riding nonstop on the way back immediately revived me. To the center of the valley took only about ten minutes, coasting almost all the way.

In winter, riding became impossible. I would often join a small group of teachers and walk to Yokota during weekends. It was fun striding through the deep snow. Once a boy teacher went off to investigate the stream running along the side of the road. He pushed the snow in with his rubber boots. I tried to imitate him and slipped into the snow, getting sopping wet. Sometimes I would walk by myself, especially the end of February to early March. Early spring, the season I was born, was my favorite time of the year. Walking over the pass quietly by myself, I could feel the power of life that had been nourished under the severe snow come into my heart. I noticed that the snow always melted first around the trees. The branches and twigs gradually turned pastel purple as a soft, warm mist condensed around them. Standing in the middle of the warm, gentle colors made me feel as if I were pushed up to the sky from the energy coming from the bottom of the valley. Early spring, with its sprouting, hidden life power, is the most glorious time of year.

In order to teach in Maki, it was necessary to live in the village. From my modest salary, I rented an upper room in a small farmhouse down the lane from the school. There was another teacher in the room next to mine. Each of us cooked for ourselves on a small charcoal stove. I ate very simply. Often the children would bring homemade mochi. They would give me an assortment of ten or fifteen pieces. Each one had a unique taste and texture. I wondered why. I realized that the soil in which the rice grew, the quality of water, and the way of pounding were slightly different for each one. This was the beginning of my understanding of food as energy.

One day in Maki, I came upon a newspaper or magazine article about Mr. Omodaka, a literary scholar. I had admired his commentaries on the *Manyōshu* in college and was eager to read about him. The article mentioned that he always ate brown rice. It was common knowledge in Japan that whole-grain rice was best for health, but for centuries in the Far East, the aristrocracy had preferred white rice. Over time it became a status symbol for other classes, too. Growing up in the countryside, we normally ate rice that had been lightly to moderately polished, from 30 percent to 70 percent.

Mr. Omodaka's poetic spirit deeply inspired me in college. The passing reference to brown rice in the article aroused my curiosity. I decided to try his way of eating. The region where I lived was divided into Great Maki and Little Maki. On the other side of the hill tower, in Little Maki, about a half hour's walk away, there was an old water-driven mill that produced excellent brown rice. One of my pupils who lived in the area volunteered to bring me five-pound bags of brown rice. I cooked it in a small clay pot with a handle on one side. The brown rice was very delicious, and I continued to make it every day for the next three years.

I also enjoyed *yakigome*, roasted rice. In the middle of

September, some grain was harvested early, roasted in the husk, and pounded. It would be eaten right from the garden like fresh corn. Roasted rice had a wonderful, nutty taste that I have missed ever since. I also liked mountain water-cress, which I had for the first time. It grew along the small mountain stream banks in Great Maki and had a strong, pungent taste and light, delicate texture.

In many ways, the three years in Maki were the most peaceful of my life. Each morning the sunrise flooded my window with radiant light, illuminating the high mountain range in the distance. By 8 A.M. the school day began with a visit by the entire class to a small shrine to pray for ancestors and the welfare of the nation. At a reunion decades later, the students recalled my earnestness. "Tomoko Sensei put her whole energy into everything she did," one former pupil noted, "even inspecting the dust on a window." "She taught us the value of hard work," another commented. "Her example inspired us in the years to come."

As the war continued, air raid drills became more frequent. People scanned the skies for the sight of B-29s flying high overhead. Concern about brothers and fathers called to distant battlefields dominated my pupils' poetry. Reading their haiku gives a unique look at the war through the eyes of ten- and eleven-year-old country girls.

Whenever draftees left to join the army, the whole village gathered to see them off. They would go by bus to Hamada or Matsue, be assigned to units, and then be posted overseas in China, Southeast Asia, or the Pacific. Parents, children, neighbors, teachers—everyone would carry red Japanese flags and wish them success and a safe return.

> The early spring sun
> Shines for the soldiers.
> Waving goodbye, we also are excited.

*

> A clump of snow
> Sits atop the hat

Of a departing soldier.

*

In a big, strong voice,
The soldiers bid farewell
To the whole village.

*

As the bus leaves,
In the swirling snow,
We cry *Banzai*!

After their departure, it would sometimes be months before families received word from the battlefield. In the early years, the fighting went in Japan's favor. In November, 1943, I wrote this poem myself.

The principal announced to my children
News of a big victory.
Outside, melting frost.

Because of government propaganda, we didn't know that such victories were hollow. After defeats in Guadalcanal, Midway, and later the Philippines, the war was already lost. But for nearly two more years, the fighting would continue and millions of more lives would be sacrificed. The fate of their loved ones far away was a constant concern.

At the morning shrine
I pray for my brother,
Forgetting the cold.

*

Although brother is not here,
At breakfast, we still set out
A dish for him at the table.

*

While gathering spruce needles,
My brother's face appeared.

*

Pounding mochi for the New Year,
I see my brother's photograph.
He looks happy, too.

The arrival of a letter or a visit was the cause of much rejoicing.

From far, far Java,
Over the ocean,
Brother's first letter came on New Year's.

*

When the soldiers returned,
We listened all night to their story
While weaving straw ropes.

*

When I saw my brother again,
He saluted me first.

But often, news from the battlefield would be sad. The
bones and ashes of dead soldiers were returned in a small box.
Families, attired in white scarves of mourning, would carry
the boxes to the cemetery for burial.

When the brave soldier came back,
We received his spirit,
And everyone cried.

*

I place a wild chrysanthemum
On the fallen soldier's grave.

There were angry poems too. One student wrote:

Looking at a map,
The hateful Americans and British so close.
Let's smash them soon,
Go to their mainlands.

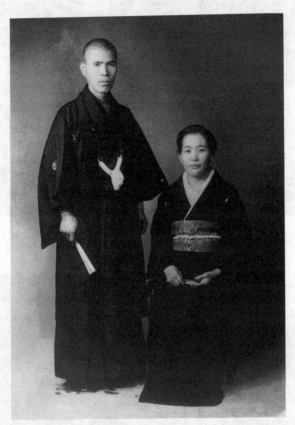

1. Banjiro and Katsue Yokoyama, Aveline's parents.

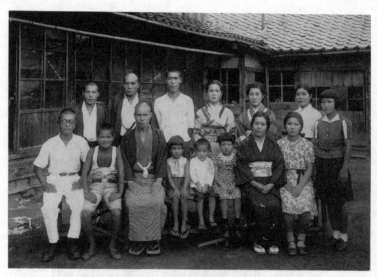

2. The Yokoyama family, mid-1940's.

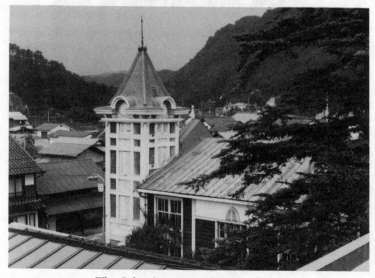

3. The Salvation Army Church in Yokota.

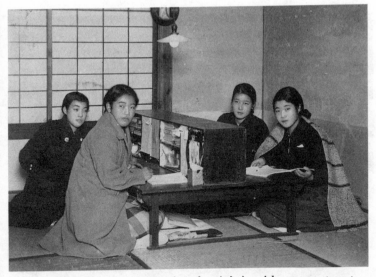

4. Aveline, at age fifteen (on the right), with roommates at Teachers' College, 1938.

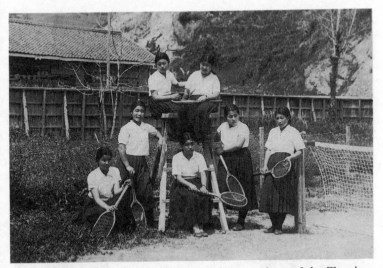

5. Aveline (second from left) and other members of the Tennis Club.

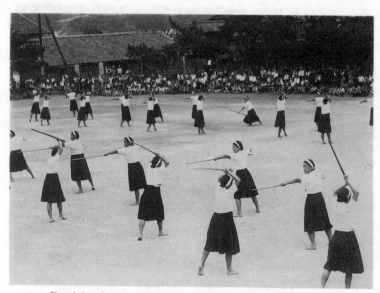

6. Participating in a ladies' sword demonstration at college.

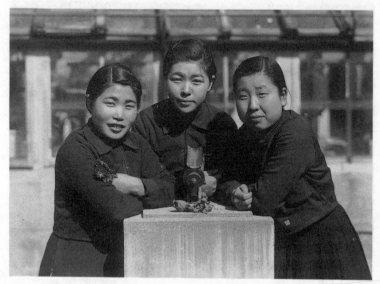

7. Aveline (left) and two graduate students, 1941.

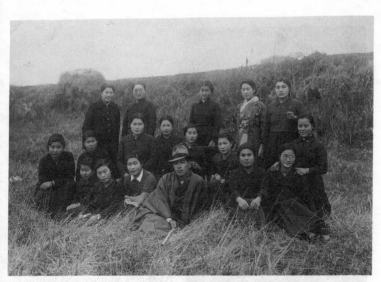

8. Mr. Tanaka, class adviser, with students, including Aveline (on his left, with white collar).

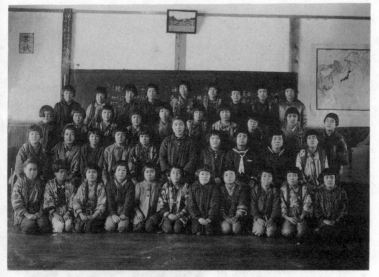

9. During World War II, Aveline (center) taught at an elementary school in the village of Maki.

70

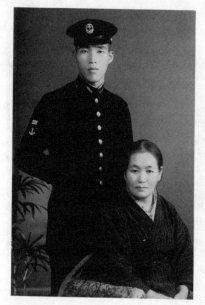

10.
Aveline's mother and brother, Makoto, who served in the Japanese Navy.

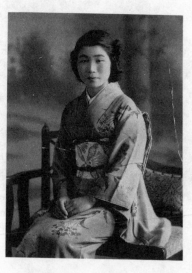

11.
Aveline in Yokota after her illness and before going to George Ohsawa's school.

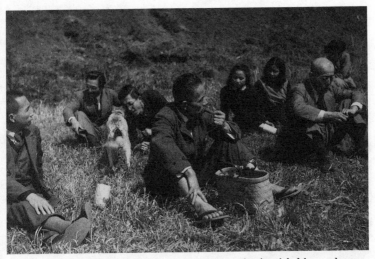

12. George Ohsawa (center, smoking a pipe) with his students.

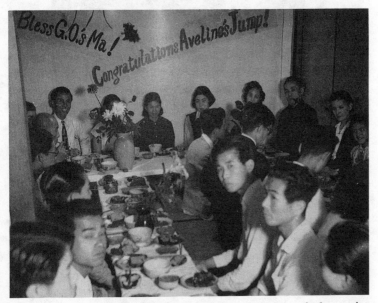

13. Aveline's farewell party at the Maison Ignoramus before going to America. (George Ohsawa, with pipe, is at top right; Lima is to the left; and Aveline is next to her.)

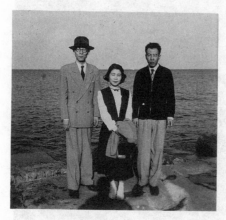

14.
Michio, Aveline, and Mr.
Shinohara (a former M.I.
student) on the Chicago
waterfront, 1951.

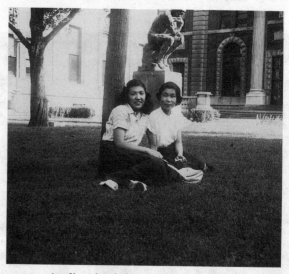

15. Aveline (right) and friend from Nagasaki
relax on Columbia University campus.

It was no wonder that the students wrote such poems because the grown-ups let the children march in the street singing slogans such as "Come out MacArthur. Fall headlong down to hell." It is a painful memory for us which we must self-reflect on deeply.

As school recessed in the summer of 1945, the war situation grew more ominous. Tokyo, the nation's capital, had been leveled in waves of saturation fire bombings. The population shrank from seven million to less than three million as surviving industries dispersed to the countryside. The Americans bombed the Japanese mainland at will, but still Izumo escaped any direct attack.

From Shanghai came word that my brother Makoto had joined a special *tokkotai*, or suicide, unit. As American forces captured Okinawa and neared the main islands, the Japanese war ministry set up a naval squadron to manually guide torpedoes toward American ships. Like the *kamikaze* pilots, the underwater torpedo men invariably lost their lives. It would be only a matter of time before Makoto received his final orders and last meal of red rice, snapper, and sake.

Meanwhile, my sister Junko had become sick while working at the plane factory in Nagoya. Mother went to take care of her. On the morning of August 6, I left Yokota to join them. The main rail line in our region ran from Hiroshima to Matsue. The train I took originated in Ochiai on the other side of the Sanyo mountains several stops after Hiroshima and two stops before Yokota. It was known as the "Zigzag Train" because of the long, back and forth track it traveled through the mountain tunnels. On the way, I heard a story that "something is happening in Hiroshima." Apparently some of those on the outskirts of Hiroshima who had been injured by the blast or seen the atomic flash managed to make it to Ochiai and board the train. They were extremely thirsty and asked for water. According to reports circulated by other passengers and the train crew, they mysteriously died after drinking the water. Nobody knew why.

One of my students at Maki had an uncle and aunt living

in Hiroshima city. As we learned later, her uncle had been
at home in the kitchen at the time of the explosion, 8:15 A.M.
Fortunately, the walls of the kitchen were made of concrete
and offered some protection from the blast. However, when
the house collapsed from the shock waves, he became trapped
under the rubble. Eventually, his wife was able to remove and
carry him to a schoolyard, which had been turned into an
emergency survival center. From there they escaped to
a nearby island where they ate rice balls. This may have protected them from radiation sickness, whose effects were not
fully appreciated for months and years later.

Nagasaki was bombed three days later, on August 9.
Details of the atomic destruction of the two cities did not
come out until many days later and then very sketchily. Like
other Japanese, our information on the course of the war came
primarily from the big national daily newspapers, the *Asahi
Shimbun* and *Mainichi Shimbun*, which were controlled by the
army, and the government radio. They ignored or minimized
the atomic bombings, which were referred to as the "gen
baku." Right up until the end, the nation had been led to
believe that the war was still winnable. Later I learned that
Kyoto had been one of the original atomic targets. Its ten
thousand Buddhist temples, Dōshisha, the Christian University, and other religious and cultural treasures had been spared
through the noble intervention of Henry Stimson, the U.S.
Secretary of War.

After changing trains in Kyoto, I reached Nagoya. Apart
from the strange rumors, the ride had been horrible enough.
There were no windows in the cars, plywood had been in-
stalled in place of glass, and the train was dangerously over-
crowded, with people hanging out the exits. In Nagoya, we
heard no further news of Hiroshima. But an unusual quiet
prevailed. As the industrial capital of Japan, Nagoya had many
war factories and had been subject to daily bombing. For the
next three or four days, the air raids mysteriously ceased.
Everyone wondered what was going on. A devil-may-care
atmosphere broke out, with much unrestrained military carous-

ing and jubilation. Some people thought the American fleet had been turned back. Others were not so sure. Inside, everyone had strange, unfamiliar feelings.

Morale in Japan was deteriorating. Despite rationing, it was hard to get decent food. Essentials such as gas, charcoal, and fabric for clothing had disappeared. Many restaurants had closed, and there was no public entertainment of any kind. Daily life was drab. The nation's leaders kept asking the people to make more sacrifices. "Desire Nothing Until Victory" was the national slogan. Under these miserable conditions, many people took out their frustration by vandalizing railroad cars and other government operations.

After attending to Junko in Nagoya, Mother and I returned a few days later to Yokota. A special radio bulletin on the morning of August 15 announced that the Emperor would address the nation. About noon, friends and neighbors gathered around our radio at home to listen. Mr. Okazaki had brought one of the first radios to Izumo province in 1931. It was a Victrola with a giant trumpet speaker. As children we often gathered to listen to it in a corner of the Okazakis' spacious house. I remember the first time, the sound was unclear, and we couldn't understand a single word.

Listening to the Emperor's speech brought back memories of those early broadcasts. The transmission on our big square set was poor. There was so much static, we could barely understand anything he said. Moreover, the possibility of Japan surrendering had not occurred to most people. Gradually, over the next few days, despite efforts by some extremists to prolong the fighting, it became clear that Japan had lost the war and that life would never be the same.

The Post-War Period

Following Japan's surrender, word came from China that Makoto was alive and well in an allied prisoner of war camp. His "human torpedo" unit had been scheduled to attack American ships on August 8, but the orders were abruptly cancelled. He would return home safely to much rejoicing. Miyako and her family were also well and returned safely from Manchuria.

However, no news of Nobue's fate was forthcoming. Along with her husband, she and her new baby were living some-where along the long northern border of Manchuria. In lafe July, the Soviet Union, which had stayed out of the Asian conflict until now attacked Japanese forces in Manchuria and seized the northernmost Kurile Islands. Eventually, over a year later, notice came from the government that Nobue and her husband had both died in the Russian attack. Their station on the Siberian border was situated at one of the main crossing points. Rather than being taken prisoners, the young couple apparently took their own lives, along with that of their child.

Our family's sadness was great. The story of strong Nobue weeping when she left Japan later seemed like a premonition. Deep inside she must have known she would never return. I inherited her Bible—a Christmas gift from the church when she was in the sixth grade—and have kept it by my side ever since.

In the immediate aftermath of the war, Japan suffered much hardship. Most major cities lay in ruins. The economy was in chaos after nearly a decade of continuous fighting. Fuel and food were scarce. Hundreds of thousands of Japanese stationed in China, Manchuria, and Southeast Asia started to return home to face lack of shelter, unemployment, and near famine. Many officers, such as one of Miyako's childhood classmates, the son of a big sake merchant in town, committed suicide at his base in Shimonoseki.

People in the countryside generally fared better than those in the city. Food was more plentiful, and they were used to a simpler way of life. Soon rice became more valuable than gold as inflation soared, first several hundred and then many thousand percent. A thriving black market flourished. City dwellers flocked to the farms and fields to exchange their kimonos, antiques, and other valuables for a handful of rice, a head of cabbage, or a bunch of radish tops.

Our remote village escaped most of the postwar suffering experienced elsewhere. There was a military storage depot at the local agricultural institute. After the war, control was temporarily lost, and some young people made off with materials. My younger brother, Kyū, a student at the institute, did not participate in the looting, which made my parents very proud. Kyū went on to graduate school and became an expert in rice cultivation. During the first several years of the postwar period, when food was scarce, he assisted farmers and helped us put in a vegetable garden. Though only a teenager, he was a very hard worker and helped our whole family through this time.

Although the rural economy held up, Father's silkscreen business continued to decline. People could no longer afford new kimonos, and restrictions on cotton meant that families had to go without new flags and banners for holidays and festivals. By the end of the war, silk was unavailable. With the arrival of American troops, Western dress became fashionable and kimonos went out of style. Makoto returned home from China and helped in the family business. But Father's health began to fail. He developed tuberculosis, and in April, 1947, he passed away. He was fifty-three. We buried his ashes in the cemetery on a mountain slope a few minutes' walk behind our home. It was a very peaceful spot, commanding a view of the entire town below, including his beloved church and bell tower.

After the war, a new minister from Shobara, a town in Hiroshima province, came to reorganize the church. For a while, the church building became a post office, and meetings were held in our home. I continued to attend Bible classes. But after the war a new translation of the scriptures appeared. Compared to the old Bible, it had no life or energy. The beautiful translation I had grown up with had been composed at the end of the Tokugawa era. No one knows by whom. But it was very poetic, like the King James Version in English, and had been used for centuries. After the new Bible came into use, I did not feel inspired to attend church.

Compared to the physical hardships, the mental and emo-

tional strains in the aftermath of the war took longer to overcome. Overnight, all values and dreams turned upside down.
As a proverb of the time put it, "One hundred million people
in a state of trauma." I remember at school when I told my
students that Japan had been defeated, one girl became paraly-
zed and couldn't move. Others cried. The shock was over-
whelming. Everyone, young and old, lost confidence in their
nation. Japan's rulers had been discredited. We couldn't
imagine what the future would bring except further disgrace
and sorrow.

The most immediate worry concerned the Americans and
what they might do. In China and Manchuria, Japanese occupation forces had been brutal, and it was only natural to
expect to be treated the same way. My pupil whose aunt and
uncle survived the atomic bombing later accompanied her
father over the mountains to Hiroshima to bring them back
to Maki to recuperate. She said she was very afraid of the
American G.I.'s who stood sentry by the temporary bridge
over the Ohta River and patrolled the obliterated city. "They
were so tall and strange looking," she recalls. "We had all
been told not to go out at night." Another girl went to
Matsue with her sister and friends. "The first time we saw
U.S. soldiers we were so afraid that we ran away."

To Japan's surprise, the Americans turned out to be friendly
and peaceful, completely unlike the foreign devils they had
been painted to be by the nation's wartime leaders. Eventually
the G.I.'s came to the countryside to see whether demilitari-
zation was being properly carried out. In Yokota and Maki,
they politely requested that all nationalist images, such as the
Imperial Rescript that had been posted in all schools, be taken
down. They also told teachers that they were no longer to take
children to the shrine in a corner of the schoolyard, where
nationalist prayers had been recited. Patriotic statues were
taken down, including those of old Ninomiya whom the
Americans understandably confused with nationalist statesmen.
The curriculum also changed. General Douglas MacArthur,
head of the American Occupation, abolished Shūshin.

"We were educated under nationalism," a classmate of mine at Teachers' College later explained. "We were taught to sacrifice our lives for the Emperor. Why did we do that? After the war, we gradually realized it wasn't right. As teachers, we became aware of the power of education. It was frightening. The arts, dancing, and singing had all been influenced by nationalism. Before we had no doubts. Now we began to question everything."

Following a Shadow

The autumn following the end of the war, I attended an educational seminar in Matsue and met a man on the train who was reorganizing the school system in Yokota. He admired my poetry and invited me to join the faculty of the new high school. In November, I left Maki, returned home, and began to teach dance, gymnastics, and Japanese language. There were few male teachers at that time, and I ended up devoting considerable time to training the high school boys in athletics. In addition to gymnastics, I taught fencing and baseball. In college I had pitched softball, but the boys enjoyed hardball, so that is what we played.

Outside the baseball diamond and classroom, I became active in the Woman's Club and Youth Club and put my energy into acting, dancing, and singing. During the Ancestors Festival in midsummer, it was customary to celebrate, and each region or province had slightly different festivities. Our club decided to organize a new program. We met and practiced upstairs in my father's workshop. My younger sister, Atsumi, and my brother, Makoto, also joined. One friend composed an official town song, another provided the lyrics, and I choreographed a folk dance to accompany it. My arrangement was a large circle dance, performed in the street and on a stage. To the clapping of hands, beating of drums, and melody of flutes, the whole town, young and old, danced all night. Like much folk art, our celebration derived from age-old rice-planting ceremonies in which the seedlings are rhythmically placed in the earth to the accompaniment of music.

I also danced to a popular love song called "Following a Shadow" by Masao Koga. The song writer had lost his true love and never married. Mr. Okazaki's son sang the song, while I performed to it. I wore a black dress with a silk scarf. It went like this:

> Every day, rain or shine, I follow your imaginary shadow.
> It is sad and painful for me even to see the moon.
> If I hold my feelings inside, the fire in my heart burns
> even stronger.
> My whole body is aflame and I weep.

> Loneliness at least released my pain.
> I take out my guitar and begin to strum.
> How long will the autumn rain continue?
> The guitar's melody is sad, and I am so sorrowful.

> Because of you, this long autumn night died in the frost.
> My life will never enjoy the flowers of spring.
> Should I live out the rest of my life
> I shall eternally follow this ephemeral romance in search
> of my love.

Our festival was a big success and drew people from around the valley. Music and art helped give meaning to life at a time when there was nothing to focus on. At shrines in the region, a dance circuit developed, and we went from one to another having a good time. I composed many dances for our young people's organization and performed some myself.

For awhile I also became active in a political campaign. There was an idealistic young candidate named Tomiyoshi Adachi. He was running for the provincial senate. He was in Nobue's class, a good athlete, and everyone knew him very well. We went all over Izumo to meetings and campaigned in the streets. He won and became the youngest senator elected.

In 1947 a new constitution had been adopted, investing ultimate power in the Japanese people rather than the Emperor and outlawing war for all time. Peace became the new universal ideal for which the young people of the future would sacrifice their lives. One of my young friends in Yokota, Mr. Suzuki, was a cadet at a naval academy just twenty miles from Hiroshima when the war ended. He later became a teacher himself. On the way home, he passed through the city's barren landscape. "It was an experience that 'went into the bone,' " he recalls, using a traditional Japanese expression. "From then on, I became deeply committed to peace."

Meanwhile, domestic relations impinged on my new found freedom and independence. Miyako embarked on a career in the church with her husband and went to Tokyo. With Nobue's death, I was the next eldest and expected to marry before my younger sisters. The war had taken a heavy toll on boys my age. About eighty percent died in battle, and many girls would never find partners. A lady minister introduced me to a young man who had just returned from serving in the Imperial army in China. He was a nice gentleman, but I wasn't the least interested in settling down at the time. One day when he came to our village, I was away. Instead, he saw Atsumi, the next oldest sister. She was tender, warm-hearted, and like Mother—and unlike me—an excellent cook. When it became clear that I was determined to remain single, the two families and the minister consulted, and one year later they were married.

My Sickness

The rootless aftermath of the war affected me deeply. I became disoriented and gradually lost confidence in my ability to teach. I visited Mr. Tanaka, my college teacher, who was now living in Kiyo, a small fishing village on the coast between Hamada and Hagi. He had just returned from Tokyo where he had been in a rest home during the last part of the war. I spent several days with him and his family at their home

near a beautiful beach. The year before Mr. Tanaka had come
to visit me in Maki. It was wintertime and deep snow blan-
keted the mountains. We walked and sometimes jogged
together the ten miles back to Yokota, and he had been impressed with my stamina and spirit. In the past Mr. Tanaka
had always been able to encourage and guide us. But now even
he was quiet, thinking deeply about what the future would
bring. He could encourage me only to persevere. Later, he
recalled of this period in my life:

> Even to Miss Yokoyama there came the time when she
> was seized with self-analysis and doubt which everyone
> experiences in the process of human growth. Yokota,
> her home town, was unusual for a country town and had
> a pretty old tradition of Christianity in Japan. Mr.
> Yokoyama, her father, was a pious Christian who stood
> in the forefront of mission work. Being brought up in
> a strict Christian family, Miss Yokoyama could not com-
> promise and escape responsibility. She fell into the doubt
> of life, and her face often showed anguish. At such times,
> she was pitiful to behold. When she came to see me, I
> gave her a hammer instead of sympathy. However, she
> never thought ill of me nor stopped communicating with
> me, perhaps because she knew my intention.

I returned home. My life energy was at an ebb. In the
summer, I resigned my teaching post after only one year
at the new high school. Shortly afterward I began to experience a sharp pain on my left side beneath the heart. By
early autumn, it had become acute, and I feared I might have
tuberculosis. TB had been the number one cause of death in
Japan since the turn of the century. From the middle of September until the following March, I remained in bed at home.
Dr. Fujiwara, the son of the co-founder of our church, super-
vised my recovery. He diagnosed my condition as pleurisy,
a serious inflammation of a membrane of the lung. According
to medical thinking, it was most often caused by a bacterial

infection, though it could be aggravated by working too hard and psychological stress. My loss of direction, Father's death, and other pressures were taking their toll.

Later, I associated my illness partly with my diet at the time. I loved eggplant. It ripened at the beginning of summer through early fall, just when my sickness began. In a four-season climate, eggplant is very weakening. Folk wisdom in Izumo advises pregnant ladies to avoid eating it, especially in the autumn. Mother grew eggplant in her garden and cooked it very beautifully. Fried, it was very crisp and delicious. I also enjoyed it pickled.

During my sickness, I was confined to the front room of the house. I lay on my futon, wrapped in warm quilts, day and night. There was too much pain to get up or move about. Lying in bed, I could see a small patch of sky through the open top half of the *shoji* screen facing the main street. On the other side, I could look into the garden. To pass the time, I composed poems. Mother and Dr. Fujiwara told me to conserve my strength and not read or write, but I kept a notebook under my pillow. From my futon, I observed that the clouds outside always passed from west to east. I called my poems "Sickbed Sketches—Poems of Clouds Passing By." My first poems went:

My whole sky—
Just one window.
Clouds appear and disappear.

*

My sky is a deep indigo.
A caravan of clouds passes by
Without stopping.

*

I look and look.
Just like the white pigs,
Fat white clouds pass by
Without sinking down.

*

With my fingers,
I make smaller and smaller circles.
But sorry, the clouds swim and float away.

*

White clouds,
Far away clouds,
Competing clouds,
I never get tired watching the whole day.

The next series of verses focused on everyday sights and sounds.

The garden is very peaceful.
At the end of the day after the doctor comes,
The deep green
Catches my eye.

The mixed sound
Of *geta* (wooden shoes) and metal.
I hear someone opening
The fish rations.

*

The red and white cosmos flower
Blossoms in the sky,
Burning out its beauty.
That is life.

*

The white cosmos flower blossoms today.
The red one may blossom tomorrow.
My pain is starting to recede.

*

I hear children describe *benitake* (red mushrooms)
Growing in a shallow valley
And whispering to each other.

By mid-October, the foliage was in its glory. Through the window to the garden, I spent countless hours watching the flowers bloom.

In the bright noontime
The cosmos flower blossoms.
The graceful petals on its head
Cannot sustain the weight of a big bee
And begin to droop.

*

In the quiet autumn rain
It grows dark.
One weak fly flits by
And catches my eye.

*

The bright, soft blossoms
Of the white ginger flower
Are born
Full of life.

*

Far, far, high in the sky,
Swallows gather together
Forming a black streak.
In a minute they are gone.

*

Sparrows flutter around
The beautiful white *gin-mokusei* flower,
Singing to themselves
As its petals fall gently down.

*

Many people pass to and fro.
But no one mentions
The beauty of this flower.

With the approach of winter, the days grew shorter and the
energy of the earth started to recede.

When the sun shines,
The cherry leaves turn bright red,
Falling against the vast sky behind.

*

When the shadows lengthen,

It becomes dark and quiet.
When the sun appears again
The cherry leaves turn bright red.

*

I can hear the sound of my pain
As my eye follows
The flight of a dragonfly.

*

The smell of sardines.
Mother bought some fish today.
How much the folks in Iwami
Enjoy making sushi.

*

When I scared a little spider
She grew smaller and smaller
Before gradually starting to move.

*

When I startled her again,
The spider became so scared
She died.

The annual Shrine Festival Day fell on November 1. I was
still not well enough to get out of bed.

Checking my temperature,
I still have a fever.
I feel sad while people in the house
Prepare for the festival.

*

The sky is a beautiful blue,
Clean and clear.
Outside I can hear the sound
Of children playing volleyball again—
Pong, pong.

A short time later, the farmers started to gather for the
Cow Market. I could watch from the window and hear the

sounds of their animals on the main street out front.

> In the beautiful autumn,
> Baby cows and horses pass by my window.
> Following their families with love and care
> With blue patterned clothing on their backs.

*

> When the days grow shorter and shorter,
> All insects in the garden
> Dance on top of the daikon and turnips,
> Bidding farewell to autumn.

*

> A *kaki* fruit rests in my hand.
> I can tell there has been frost
> On the ground this morning
> Because I feel cold when I hold it.

*

> My left shoulder feels weak.
> The pain continues.
> It's already the middle of November.

As winter arrived, the only flowers to cheer me were those that grew indoors. One day I was even able to stand up and peek out into the street.

> A yellow chrysanthemum
> Blossoms in a pot,
> As the sunshine becomes stronger
> From time to time.

*

> The wind stops,
> And a mixture of rain and snow comes.
> One yellow chrysanthemum lies in the road.
> Who left it there?

A visit of schoolchildren from the mountains helped to brighten the long winter.

In pain and sorrow,
I am watching their wet sneakers,
As my pupils from Maki leave.
They keep turning back to wave goodbye,
Disappearing along the snowy road.

*

The line of mountains in the distance
Is so beautiful and soft.
Beyond lies the village of Maki.
I drink in the memories.

In Yokota, spring usually arrived at the end of February,
the season I was born. The first wild grasses began to peek
through the snow. As the weather changed, I felt new energy
and life stir within me.

Struggling with sickness,
The long winter now past,
I hold the budding energy
Of spring close to my heart.

*

As I change my sleeping position,
The pain disappears
And my joy increases.

*

My father has passed away.
Spring has returned again
To my homeland after another year.
I feel sad when I see Mother's white hair increase.

*

Our rabbit grows skinny and dies.
We feel very sad.
The snowy days of winter
Fade into our memories.

In March the last symptoms of my sickness left. With each
new day, I grew stronger in body and spirit.

The swallows dance and sparrows sing.
The clouds float back and forth.
Day by day spring becomes full
In my window.

After my recovery, I presented my little handmade book of
poems to Dr. Fujiwara. I was grateful for his kindness and
help during my illness. But it was nature that had healed me.
In my renewed faith in the sky and earth and all the manifestations of life around me, I realized that dying for one's
country could no longer be an ideal. The world was now one.
From now on, I would devote my life to world peace and
harmony.

In the autumn I resumed teaching at the local kindergarten as a full-time substitute. I still didn't know how I
would be able to realize my new dream. During the following
year, Mitsuko Yodono, the tennis star, sent me some world
government literature from Tokyo. Efforts to strengthen the
newly formed United Nations and prevent a worldwide nuclear
war caught my imagination. But I was shocked by the poor
quality of the newspaper and its strong, pushy tone.

Like Nobue, Mitsuko and her family had been stationed
along the Siberian border in Manchuria at the end of the war.
When the Russians attacked, they fled and wandered through
the desolate region for months with other refugees. All but
one of her children died from hunger or sickness. The hardships became so great that she lost the power to cry. Eventually she made it back to Japan with one son.

In Yokota, we became close friends. For a while, she helped
an associate establish a Western-style sewing school which
became very successful. Then she went to Tokyo and got a
job with a big insurance company, Chiyoda-Seimei, where
her brother and sister-in-law worked. Pretty soon, Mitsuko
held the sales record.

Returning to Yokota on New Year's Day 1950, Mitsuko
spoke at a small meeting I arranged at the Women's Club in
the high school. She was accompanied by a colleague, Minoru

Fukumoto. They explained that lasting world peace began with each individual. Unlike the world government literature she had sent earlier, their words were convincing and touched my heart. Responding to my enthusiasm, Mitsuko invited me to come to Tokyo and meet her wonderful new teacher. His name was George Ohsawa.

5: Life at Maison Ignoramus

Asta: I imagine he was subject to the law of
   change. . . .
Borgheim: What a stupid law that must be!
   Anyway, I don't believe in it.
Asta: You might have to, someday.
                              —Ibsen, *Little Eyolf*

THE MORNING of February 2, 1950, Mt. Torikami, where the eight-headed dragon had lived, was under a quilt of deep snow. The Hi or Chopstick River, which was said to have turned red with the serpent's blood when Susa-no-wo slew it, was iced over. I would look back on the day I left home to study macrobiotics as the turning point of my life. From Yokota, the train ride to Tokyo took altogether about twenty hours. From Kyoto, I changed to the Tokaido line, which ran along the picturesque stretch of road immortalized by Hokusai in fifty-four beautiful woodcuts, and then to the Toyoko line. In Yokohama I changed to the Tokyo spur. I arrived in Hiyoshi, the suburb where George Ohsawa's dormitory was located, before the sun was up. Hiyoshi means "Lucky Day." At the deserted train platform, a sign with the station name caught my eye. Just before sunrise, Hiyoshi seemed a particularly auspicious destination.

Mitsuko Yodono had sent me directions to the dormitory. I followed her description, listening to the echo of my own footsteps on the wet pavement. From the station, I walked for about ten minutes up the center of the main road, turning right at the local police station. There were beautiful houses on both sides of the street with lovely ornamental bushes sprinkled with light snow. Several blocks further, I came across a simple house surrounded by a hedge. There was an old plum tree in the yard with outstretched, snowy branches. Next to it was a two-storied building which did not match the main house. It had a big sign on the roof. Even in the dark I could read its characters: *Sekai Seifu* (Student World Government Association). I had been busy preparing for my visit since New Year's. Events of the last month passed through my mind as I neared the end of my journey.

Before Mitsuko's talk to the Women's Club, I had never thought about food itself as the shaper of life, health, and peace. I had eaten brown rice for several years while teaching in the mountains. But I also took many things that were not part of the macrobiotic diet.

From the first or second grade, I remembered receiving candy on special occasions and had heard the name chocolate. Growing up, we didn't have much sugar, and what we had was very expensive. It was brown, measured out in tiny spoons, and eaten very infrequently. White sugar was extremely rare. We never ate it at home, but my mother would sometimes prepare a small package of white sugar as a gift for someone. During the war, sugar virtually disappeared, but with the arrival of the G.I.'s, it came back. Suddenly there were tons of sugar available. It was processed in small cubes and distributed free or at very low cost in big buckets as part of the relief effort. Bakery stores opened for the first time after the war, and highly refined Western-style bread, biscuits, and pastries also became popular.

Like most Japanese, I did not eat very much meat, poultry, or eggs and consumed no dairy food. But at college, fresh high-quality fish and seafood were plentiful, and I ate them whenever they were served in the dormitory. In Izumo, I also enjoyed a wide variety of wild foods including ferns, mushrooms, and other large, soft, primitive plants which, taken in excess, macrobiotic theory associated with leprosy and other rare diseases that afflicted mountain people. Among tropical fruits and vegetables, I enjoyed juicy ripe persimmons and succulent eggplants. Looking back, I started to think that these foods may have caused my illness as well as contributed to my loss of direction.

Except in Maki when I lived in the farmhouse, I had never really cooked before. My knowledge was very limited. The wife of the doctor across the street from our home in Yokota began giving classes in modern cooking, featuring butter, wheat flour, sauces, and dressings. I was taking classes with her at the time Mitsuko spoke. After hearing about macrobiotics, I decided to change completely my way of eating. That very day, New Year's, I made up my mind. I decided to go to Tokyo and meet George Ohsawa.

Before, I had not been at all impressed with Ohsawa's articles in the World Government newspaper Mitsuko had sent me. His language was coarse, strident, and mocking. He delighted in slang and made-up words. The paper itself was clumsily designed and printed and gave the feeling of a communist, underground publication. But after her speech, I sensed he knew something that I never studied. I didn't know what, but I was determined to find out.

My family laughed when I started to eat simple brown rice and miso soup because I had just started taking modern, Western-style cooking classes. Fortunately, I didn't have a husband or family to take care of and was free to leave. I sent in my resignation to school and on January 20 taught my last class. I spent the next ten days preparing to leave, selling my kimono and umbrella to pay for my train ticket.

The low white stucco main house was situated next to the building with the World Government sign. In a shuttered room facing the garden, a solitary lamp cast a dim light. I later learned it was George Ohsawa's room. He usually slept only a few hours at night, rising at 2 A.M. He would enjoy the peace and quiet of the early hours to read and write until the rest of the household awoke at 7. Not wanting to disturb those sleeping inside, I waited by the side of the house for an hour or two, counting the remaining stars in the sky. While standing there, I remembered that I hadn't washed up in the train and scooped up some lightly lying snow from the ground to scrub my face. Unknown to me, someone inside the house was watching from a window. Ohsawa was notorious for his spartan discipline, and he never wore socks in the house, even in the coldest days of winter. Cleaning my face in the snow immediately earned me the reputation for being very yang—bold, fearless, and immune to the elements.

As the sky grew light, I heard someone drawing water from a well with a bucket and the sound of voices in the house. I went around to the kitchen and opened a wooden wicker door. A tall, vigorous lady came out. "We are expecting you, Tomoko-san," she said. "Mitsuko told us about you. We are happy you have come."

I had arrived via the back entrance. A twisted pine tree jutted out by a gate, marking the main approach. On top of the gate, in the evergreen branches, a sign in French proclaimed the name of the school: *La Maison Ignoramus* (the House of Ignorance). I was so foolish I didn't even see the sign for several months, continuing to come and go the back way. In the United States, anyone who put such signs in front of their house and kept a dormitory inside would have been harassed by neighbors and not been allowed to stay very long. And what was worse, the scattered loud grace that issued from the front room every morning sounded like a cracked bell and could be heard next door. But fortunately, Japanese are very accepting, and the neighbors never complained.

The purpose of the Maison Ignoramus was to become free —free of fear, free of doubt, free of anger and hatred, free of disease. The goal was to be free of everything that was preventing us from realizing our true selves and infinite health, happiness, and peace. In Ohsawa's own case, the road to freedom had not been easy. He was born in 1893 in a suburb of Kyoto to parents of samurai descent and was known originally as Yukikazu Sakurazawa. When Yukikazu was six years old, his father summarily divorced his mother, leaving her to bring up two small boys alone. In his teenage years, both his mother and brother died of tuberculosis. At age eighteen, Yukikazu also came down with the dread disease.

Doctors told him there was nothing that could be done and he would probably die.

One day, at a second-hand bookstore in Kyoto, Yukikazu came across a small book, *The Curative Method by Diet*, by Sagen Ishizuka, M.D. Ishizuka, a former veterinarian and army doctor, believed that departure from Japan's traditional diet and reliance on refined foods underlay the epidemic of tuberculosis and other diseases of modern society. Known as Dr. Miso Soup and Dr. Daikon, Ishizuka ran a medical clinic in Tokyo, attracting thousands of patients. Young Yukikazu tried his regimen of brown rice, miso soup, cooked vegetables, beans, and seaweed, and the symptoms of tuberculosis disappeared, never to return. From that time on, Yukikazu devoted his life to spreading the teachings of the Shoku-Yo Kai (Cure by Food Society) that Ishizuka's supporters founded in 1908. He quickly became the dominant figure in the movement, marrying Ishizuka's scientific-medical principles with the traditional philosophy of the East—Vedanta, Buddhism, and especially the yin/yang teachings of Lao Tzu and Confucius.

In the late 1920s and 1930s, Sakurazawa spent about ten years living in Paris, teaching Oriental medicine and philosophy as well as Jūdo, haiku composition, and flower arrangement. In France, he adopted the pen name Jean G. Ohsawa and began to write the first of several hundred books, articles, and pamphlets on diet, health, and society. Later he shortened it to just George Ohsawa. He met many influential Western authors and scientists and plunged into studies of literature, religion, chemistry, and even miniature aircraft design. Returning to Japan as the situation in Manchuria and China intensified, he alternately supported and opposed Japan's military buildup. From his long experience abroad, he knew that it would be foolhardy for Japan to get into a war with the West. For writing a book predicting Japan's defeat by the United States and organizing other anti-government activities, he spent the last years of the war in prison under sentence of death.

Liberated by the Americans, he devoted his energies after the war to the world government movement as did many other great men such as Einstein, Nehru, and Bertrand Russell. However, to end the arms race and achieve lasting peace, Ohsawa felt that society must return to a more natural, organic way of farming and eating. He taught that world government did not begin at the top with political changes. It began at the bottom with the recovery of the health and happiness of each individual, family, and community.

I first met this remarkable man a few days after my arrival in Hiyoshi. I didn't have any money and spent the first couple of days in Tokyo looking for a job. My first evening at dinner, he came to the table and distributed copies of *Life*, *Time*, *Paris-Match*, and other magazines and books from around the world. His dress and manner were very casual, not at all like a regular teacher. He wore a sports jacket, a cotton shirt open at the neck, and was puffing on a pipe. "Hello, what have you been doing today?" he would ask someone with a broad grin. "What do you think of this?" he would say to another, pointing to a headline or article in a magazine. His speech was very interesting, full of current affairs, skipping from events in Japan to the United States, Europe, and around the world. I realized I was in the presence of someone very unusual. His refined and somewhat Westernized behavior was not like that which could be scornfully called "Western Copy" by other Japanese but was always full of wit and lovable childishness in addition to breadth and depth. I had never heard such stimulating, global conversation before. It was a pattern that would continue at meals and lectures. He would never teach directly about food or sickness, just world government and world structure. If a question about diet or personal health came up, he would answer it in just one or two words and then put it aside.

As the conversation continued, I became vaguely aware that everyone at the table had suddenly become very serious. He had begun to chide some of the students for their replies to his off-handed questions. Heads were down in the looking-

scared posture. Directly across from him, at the other end of
the table, my face was still up looking naively ahead.

"Oh, you are the newcomer, aren't you?" he said with
a penetrating stare through his black horn-rimmed glasses.

"Yes, I've just come from the country of Izumo," I replied.

"The letter you sent was a real waste of paper," he said
sternly. "Next time, use only one sheet."

I had sent him a letter from Yokota, informing him that
I would like to visit Hiyoshi and meet him. It had been written on several sheets of elegant stationary in a large, formal
calligraphic hand with beautiful brushstrokes. Later I learned
that he was a fanatic about paper. To a perpetually penniless
writer and publisher like Ohsawa, paper and ink were like
blood. They had often been scarce and expensive. Over the
years he acquired the habit of writing his manuscripts on the
inside of old envelopes, on the back of grocery lists or laundry
slips, and anything else that could be reused. He wrote in the
smallest possible hand, often running to the edge of the sheet
without leaving room for margins.

"What are you going to do?" he asked.

"I'm looking for work to survive," I replied.

He then asked the other students to evaluate my condition
using the methods of traditional Oriental visual diagnosis they
had learned in his lectures. The general conclusion was that
my face was red from eating too much persimmon. He later
dubbed me "the girl from the Izumo mountains with a face
as red as a monkey's rump" because of my fondness for this
fruit. I blushed in embarrassment but inside had to admit they
had diagnosed correctly.

I soon learned that there were three qualifications for the
Maison Ignoramus. The student of life must have a dream,
poetry, and passion. George Ohsawa loved these three words
above all others. "You have to live in these three worlds,"
he continually told us. "Otherwise, you're dead." His dream
of world government and world peace through peaceful
biological change permeated every conversation and action.

His every comment and gesture reverberated with poetry and passion.

The young people he attracted to the school were just the opposite. In truth they were far from the adventurous world of dreams, poems, and passion. My first impression of my fellow students was how unkempt and dirty they were. Students in Japan, whether in a public or private school, a classroom or a martial arts dōjō, customarily wore the same uniform and prided themselves on being neat and clean. The boys sported sweaty, sloppy, indistinguishable school uniforms, and the girls with shabby clothes and worn-out shoes and wooden clogs had no sense of style or fashion. I wondered if they had ever been taught how to take care of themselves. To normal Japanese eyes, M.I. dress standards were very shocking.

I gradually realized that this casual attire was another form of George Ohsawa's social teaching. During the war, everyone not only thought alike but they dressed alike. The military government censored everything, and the country was blind to world affairs. In this era of conformity, George Ohsawa desperately wanted to tell people, even just one or two individuals, the truth of a much wider world. He found that by shocking people with unconventional dress, language, and actions he could get their attention. Dispensing with Japanese formalities was a bold way to make a point. Instead of addressing him as *Sensei*, or Master, in the traditional manner and bowing, he had us greet him as Papa or George in the Western style and shake hands or embrace.

One of the things George Ohsawa particularly admired about the Americans was their punctuality and sharpness. When he asked a question, he expected an immediate answer. Whether it was a simple request or a profound inquiry —"What is faith?" or "What is love?"—he wanted a quick, preferably poetic and passionate reply. To realize his dream, he knew that time was at a premium. World government and world peace would not be realized by a world of slow thinkers. In the Japanese countryside, we observed a slower and more leisurely pace. Adjusting to Ohsawa's standards of promptness and efficiency took some getting used to.

Another common source of censure was daily reports.
George Ohsawa expected all students to submit to him written
comments on what they had learned or were thinking. The
first time I submitted a note, it came back with a big X
scrawled across it in pen. In places there were holes in the
paper, showing he had used his whole strength. I was shocked.
I exclaimed to one of the girls, "Never before in my whole
life have I received such a grade, and besides, there are holes
in the paper!"

I wondered how my paper could be so much in error. I told
my friend that I had only recorded simply and sincerely my
feelings upon entering the school and had given this to him.
I had written: "When one goes to a Christian church, it is
said that everyone is a 'child of sin,' and one begins to feel
attacked by this word 'sin' which is so often and randomly
used. Here, in the same way, everything is referred to in
terms of yin and yang. In those words, Yin and Yang, there
is something of the bad odor of organized religion."

Fortunately, I did not let George Ohsawa's scoldings or
criticisms disturb me. Being from the cloud-swept mountains,
I was used to sudden, unpredictable changes in the weather.
Beneath his dragonlike exterior, I could always feel his warm
heart. I sensed that he deliberately used humorous and childish
ways to educate us. I came to realize that yin and yang really
are the compass for a life of health and happiness. George
Ohsawa's attitude toward me also softened. He later told
students that it was one of his joys to see my writings.

Everyone at Maison Ignoramus was known by a Western
name. In addition to our unique looks, our new names were
another very surprising and fantastic thing which ordinary
Japanese people would not have understood at the time.
George Ohsawa selected them from the names of great people
and heroes who were born in the same month as his students.
They became known as P.U. names after the abbreviation
for "Principe Unique," by which he referred to the teachings
of yin and yang in French. Naming his students in this way
seemed to be an expression of George's ardent wish that all
of his students travel abroad. He wanted to let us know the

world situation in order to rescue the Japanese people blind-folded by militarism and the vortex of defeat.

When I arrived, only one person didn't have a P.U. name, Mr. Nagata. With black-framed glasses and a thick beard, he looked like a run-down communist or socialist. One day, while we sat on the thin straw mats listening to the morning lecture around a long, slender table as usual, Mr. Nagata all of a sudden flared up and started yelling and hitting the table. We were all scared with his ferocity. George Ohsawa collected his books and quickly hurried out of the room to his study. Mr. Nagata left and never came back.

There was a young college student named Mash. Despite his squalid appearance, he was very smart. He came from Yamanashi province, on the back side of Mt. Fuji, the same area where Lima, George's wife, was born. Another ragtag-looking boy was known as Zelman. He worked for a printing company, and his hands were always black and greasy. His eyes were bloodshot, and he shivered as if cold. About the same time I arrived, two brothers came from Kyushu, Japan's southernmost island. The elder, Alcan Yamaguchi, left his job as a high school teacher to come and help edit World Government publications. A hard worker, he always sat at George Ohsawa's right hand during lectures. In Japanese, his name Alcan meant "he who does not walk." Ohsawa would scold him humorously to increase his speed and quickness, "Please walk quickly. Why you don't 'Alcan,' Alcan?" The younger brother, Seigo, was called Rudolf, and was much bigger and more energetic. He looked like a wolf howling at the moon. I thought that his swaggering was meant to get the attention of the girls. Rudolf later became an eighth rank Aikido master with many disciples.

The one normal dresser among the boys was named Raphael. He was the son of a doctor. There was a conservative, but absent-minded dreamer known as Libéral. He had a lot of nervous energy and was hoping to invent something like George Ohsawa, whose own scientific experiments had resulted in several inventions, both practical and impractical. On his

window ledge, the master of the household kept assorted
bottles and beakers. It was his dream to invent a sugarless
soft drink to compete with Coca-Cola, which had conquered
Japan after the war. Whether or not Libéral invented anything,
he is still teaching macrobiotics in Osaka. There was a quiet
boy named Parfait (French for "Perfected"). He was very
artistic. Also, Herman Aihara, who is now teaching in California, was staying there for two weeks that spring. He was
so quiet I didn't realize he was present. Only many years later
at a gathering in the United States did I learn our stays at
the dormitory had coincided.

The boy whom I got to know best was named Abe in honor
of Abraham Lincoln, one of George Ohsawa's American heroes.
He was young, only fourteen when he first came to the dormitory. As a boy he had read Alexis Carrel's *Man the Unknown*,
a book by a famous French scientist that George Ohsawa had
translated in the late 1930s. Inspired by Ohsawa's vision of
a harmonious society, he came to Hiyoshi several years after
the war.

Young and in good health, Abe was always binging. George
Ohsawa nicknamed him Seven Times Abe because once he
devoured seven small loaves of French bread in one sitting.
Abe was often naughty, pulling pranks and practical jokes,
but he could do what others couldn't. His accomplishments
included fasting for forty days. Once when the G.I.'s came to
Yokohama, they advertised for a typist. Abe applied, even
though he had never touched a typewriter. He was penniless,
wearing poor straw sandals at the time. He got the job and
said that the secret of his success was fasting for eight days.
His feat was known ever after as the 8th Day Fasting Miracle.
He stayed at Hiyoshi altogether six years, longer than anyone
else. Serving as George Ohsawa's secretary for some of the
time, he would go off in search of volumes by Thoreau,
Whitman, and other authors and poets Ohsawa asked for to
use in lectures or to have the students translate into Japanese.

There was another pair of brothers, the Satos. The younger
was also known as Abe, the elder as Roman. Their parents

owned a printing shop in Tokyo where *Le Compas*, George Ohsawa's magazine, was printed. They visited the M.I., staying often for dinner and evening lectures. When Ohsawa became angry, they disappeared just before the thunderbolt. This behavior earned Roman the nickname Irregular Off-Track Train. (Today he is a very successful businessman in New York City.)

Mitsuko's son was living at the dormitory at the time. He was about ten years old and the only one of her children to survive the ordeal in Manchuria. The father had subsequently passed away, so he and his mother, whose P.U. name was Yura, were all that remained of the original family. Because of his lively activity, George Ohsawa named him Yo-Yo, and his beautiful, childish voice made the school very bright. He is now living in Brazil.

There was another young boy, about thirteen, named Juste, and one with a cute round face and light footsteps named Tamura. Later Juste and I teamed up to sell World Government newspapers together. Tamura is now an Aikido master in Marseilles, in the south of France. George Ohsawa used Yo-Yo and Juste as models for a children's book, *Jack and Yo-Yo in Alice-Land*. Parfait did the drawings under Ohsawa's instructions. It chronicled the adventures of two youngsters who visited the country of Erewhon, the land of nowhere and no war, and learned about the Unique Principle. Samuel Butler's utopian romance, *Erewhon*, was one of George Ohsawa's favorite books. He often talked about it in his lectures. We came to admire the imaginary realm where the sick were sent to jail for violating the order of nature and criminals were sent to the hospital and given proper food to get well.

Many of the other boys I knew only by name such as Pascal, Augustine, Anatole, and André. They were living in the boys' dormitory or had already left for Europe or America when I arrived, but George Ohsawa spoke of them constantly. The boys at M.I. lived together on the first floor of the World Government building. Above them, on the second floor were the editorial offices for *Le Compas* and the World Government newspaper, which George Ohsawa would usually reach by ascending the stairway two or three steps at a time. The boys' quarters resembled a barracks or ship with rows of bunk beds. The boys' dormitory was known by the initials W.G. George would often chastise them, "Your room is not W.G., it's W.C. It is smelly, dirty, and bad. You must clean it up."

The girls at M.I. slept in the main house. The most central girl was known as Darbin like Deena Darbin, the famous orchestra singer. She was tall, very different in appearance from her namesake whom I knew from the movies during my college time. She was the one who welcomed me the first morning. As cook, she managed the kitchen and ran it strictly like a Zen monastery. If anything unpleasant happened during the day, George Ohsawa accused the kitchen. In his view, the cook was the first one responsible for the health and harmony of the entire household. Darbin had great passion and was a hard worker. I felt like I had known her all my life and that we understood one another heart to heart. In Japanese, *Dobin* means "ceramic tea kettle," and she adopted this "Broken Dobin" (Darbin) as her nickname. She sometimes sang when she was happy, but she was invariably off key. When we heard her singing, like a broken tea kettle, it was a sign that everything was all right. Papa was in a good mood, and everyone was very happy.

Meals were very simple, consisting of brown rice, miso soup, and some vegetables, well cooked and delicious. For me there was no problem staying on the diet. Yet for others, there was a tendency to binge. Those who went out and ate unhealthy things didn't want to be in the lecture room and would eat well for two or three days before attending. George Ohsawa never mentioned a person's day-to-day condition or way of eating. But he would always bring up something else and scold the person. In this way he taught people to relate cause and effect.

Helping Darbin in the kitchen most was Judy, a strong, earnest young woman born in the northern snow country. She had studied to become a nurse. At age nineteen, she came

down with tuberculosis and went to many hospitals in search
of a cure. The chief doctor of her local clinic had heard of
George Ohsawa and suggested that brown rice and miso soup
might be of some help. She read some books by Ohsawa the
doctor lent her. Her whole family opposed macrobiotics, but
Judy told them she didn't mind trying because nothing else
had worked. In three months, her condition improved, and
the depression of the last three years started to lift. A positive, future dream of happiness replaced the very dark feelings
of the past. Later she met George Ohsawa at a lecture, and he
invited her to come and study with him. After passing her
nursing test, she came to Myorenji, where he lived prior to
moving to Hiyoshi. There were two other students studying
with him at the time, including young Abe.

In the M.I. kitchen, Judy handled consultations and recipes
for sick people. Ohsawa was beseiged with patients seeking
relief for their ailments. He entrusted the preparation of
special dishes and traditional home remedies to Judy, mindful
of her nursing background. Unlike most present-day macrobiotic counselors, George Ohsawa would only see a person
once. He felt that after he had diagnosed a condition and explained the proper remedy, it was the individual's responsibility to get well. Judy put her whole effort into following
his instructions but made many mistakes and was scolded
bitterly. I sometimes saw her crying and admired her perseverance. At such times, she was as tenacious as a person
from the Hokuriku area.

Lima, George Ohsawa's beautiful wife, also helped in the
kitchen but did not do the cooking. She was very quiet and
dressed stylishly, wearing fancy blouses and long black, grey,
or navy blue skirts. Unlike everyone else who knelt on the
tatami mats with legs tucked up underneath, she always sat
sideways. The dining room was a step down from the tatami
room, and she often sat on the top step. After an unhappy
first marriage, she had begun studying with George Ohsawa
shortly before the war. He gave her the name Lima. Soon
they started living together and eventually married.

George Ohsawa instructed Lima in many things, and she followed his lead. From time to time, she relayed messages from him to the students. She also helped with bookkeeping and writing. We could feel that she was also scolded by her husband. At the time I studied there, George was fifty-seven and she was fifty-two. In later years, we became much closer. She told many stories about him such as how he would occasionally throw away whole trays of food she had cooked when he was in a bad mood. She attributed his enormous energy and violent outbursts to having taken so much salt in his younger years. He found that excessive amounts of salt kept him awake and he could get by with only four hours of sleep each night. George Ohsawa's later writings reflected this extreme use of salt. The first generation of European and American macrobiotic friends who followed his recipes acquired a reputation for zealous behavior.

From the southernmost part of the country, Kagoshima, came a girl we called Mary. She looked smart and accomplished and gave the impression of understanding but her comprehension wasn't really too deep. Another girl, Bertha, beautiful but out of focus, came to Hiyoshi from a mental hospital. From Hiroshima came a survivor of the atomic-bomb we called Sidonie, and from Nagasaki came the daughter of a rich family, Anne. She was one of the best-natured persons but looked older than her age because of round shoulders. From the northernmost island of Hokkaido hailed Agnes, whose bright red cheeks reminded me of an apple.

A very humble girl named Childe arrived from Fukuoka after hearing George Ohsawa lecture there. She had a history of heart trouble and was very weak. She had read many of Ohsawa's books and could quote entire passages by heart. Childe stayed in Hiyoshi for three years, and her mother also became macrobiotic.

My closest girlfriend was Bernadette. A beautiful art student, she had come across one of George Ohsawa's books in grammar school and liked the way he unified modern science and Oriental philosophy. Her sister suffered from spinal meningitis and started eating brown rice after reading about macrobiotics. The sister began to get well, but didn't really understand how to balance her meals with yin and yang. Over Bernadette's repeated objections, she ate melons, sugarcane, mushrooms, vinegar, and other strong yin foods. Her heart expanded, the doctor injected some medications, and she died. Bernadette understood the cause of death, but no one believed it.

After the war, she attended a seminar given by George Ohsawa and came to Hiyoshi to study. Her family was very wealthy and opposed her plan. At home, Bernadette had never done any housework or cleaning. At the M.I. Ohsawa put her in charge of cleaning the bathrooms. We became close friends and dreamed of taking a world trip together. She would draw and I would write.

Bernadette and I together decided to study Aikido. I would wake up early and leave before dawn to study with Morihei Uyeshiba, the founder of Aikido, at the main hall of his dōjō in the Shinjuku section of Tokyo. Bernadette had already returned to living at home, so we met together at Shinjuku Station. Since I liked archery, long-handled sword, and gymnastics, I was fascinated with this martial art and its spiral motions. Mr. Uyeshiba was very short, but he was just like a big tree, standing straight so that nobody could move him. Five or six young men in the class tried to push him aside, but he remained quietly rooted to the earth. I was amazed.

Aikido classes started at 5 A.M., and I would be back by 7 for clean-up and breakfast and went about my work as if nothing had happened. Eventually my secret reached George Ohsawa's ears. Stopping his writing for a moment, he gave me a glance over his dark glasses and said, "It is good to practice Aikido. But why don't you graduate from Shokuyō (macrobiotics) first?"

I was shocked. Shrinking back a little, I said, "Yes, I will." From that day on, I gave up going to Shinjuku to practice.

In truth, Ohsawa really appreciated the spirit of Sensei

Uyeshiba's teachings and one spring day invited him to teach us. Mr. Ohsawa arranged for us to study Aikido with him at the nearby workplace of a Mr. Okada. His factory had an extra room, and once or twice a week all of us girls and boys, as well as Lima, would practice the martial arts there. Ohsawa's students were later the first to bring Aikido to France.

Though I loved sports and gymnastics, I never kept up my Aikido studies. Many years later, visiting our home in New York, George Ohsawa rebuked me, "If you had continued Aikido, you could have been able to support Michio now."

George Ohsawa later wrote to Mr. Uyeshiba recommending that he take Bernadette as a regular student. She went to study with him and became very happy. Later, she enrolled in art school and received a scholarship to study in Italy, where she stayed eight years. George Ohsawa loved to tell the story of how once in an Aikido demonstration (she had reached the third rank by then), she bested a Swiss-Italian border guard. She went on to become a famous sculptor, and under her Japanese name, Uka Onoda, has exhibited beautiful, spirallic bronze compositions of angels and dancers around the world.

Today Bernadette has an art studio in Tokyo and still studies Aikido with an eighty-three-year-old Aikido master. Looking back on her studies at that period, she reflects, "Everyone thinks that the spirit is inside the body. But George Ohsawa said that the body is in the spirit. That impressed me. As an artist, Aikido interested me as a study of moving *ki*. My practice of Aikido made it much easier to understand macrobiotics. Food is really *ki* or spirit."

From nearby my home prefecture there was a sixteen-year-old high school girl whose P.U. name was Aida. She became macrobiotic following the example of her mother and cousin. Aida was very pretty, smart, and dutiful. George Ohsawa thought highly of her and wanted her to go abroad to America, but she returned home to take care of her mother. Later she went to Marseilles, and George Ohsawa invited her to Paris when he came to lecture. Abe, Ohsawa's young secretary, had become attracted to Aida and took her to Germany instead, where they eventually married. For eloping without permission, they incurred George Ohsawa's wrathful silence for three years. Settling in Dusseldorf, Abe and Aida Nakamura have taught macrobiotics together in Germany for the last nearly thirty years.

From Yonago, the coastal city in Izumo, there was a girl named Janne. Zelman's mother, Simone, also moved to Hiyoshi to study along with her son. Many people came and went over the year, including visitors. The summer before I arrived, Norman Cousins, leader of the world government movement in the United States and editor of the *Saturday Review of Literature*, visited the M.I. On a trip to Japan, he met several of George Ohsawa's disciples fasting in front of the peace tower in Hiroshima. They told him about the Student World Government Association, and on his way back he stopped in Hiyoshi, talking with George Ohsawa. I don't know whether or not he understood the name of the school, Maison Ignoramus. Before he entered the house, I was told he stood by the gate looking up at the name for some time.

True to my wild boar nature, I didn't know that everyone received his or her P.U. name from George Ohsawa. When I arrived, I selected a new name for myself. I called myself Asta after a character in Ibsen's play, *Little Eyolf*, which was translated in Japanese as *The Water Lily*. It was a story of a step-brother and sister who fell in love and couldn't marry, only to separate and find out later that they were not related. I had read the play toward the end of my study in college, and its beauty captured my heart. When George Ohsawa pronounced my new name gently with a French accent, it sounded good. But when my friends called it, it sounded like the name of a cheap aspirin. I would probably still be known as Asta today except for an amusing series of events. It came about in this way.

There was a small extended house next to the World Government building where George Ohsawa's library was

kept and where macrobiotic books and magazines were ware-
housed. One day George was working there, and I was as-
sisting him. He asked me to get something to cut with. I
spontaneously turned and ran out, returning in minutes with
an axe which was outside by the wood in the front yard. He
was shocked. He stopped tying the books and looked at me
slowly from head to toe a couple times. Then he said very
slowly, "That is for cutting wood. We don't use an axe in
a tatami room."

"Of course, I understand," I explained.

I dejectedly went out to get some scissors. But after that
he always called me *Masakari*, which is Japanese for The Axe.

Our daily meals at the M.I. were pretty simple, with soup
and one vegetable dish besides brown rice. Once a month we
had a party to celebrate all the birthdays of the month at the
school. Many guests from outside came to share in a beautiful
birthday cake and other festive foods prepared by Darbin.
For parties the sliding door between the two front rooms next
to the big tatami room was taken out to accommodate the
visitors. On these occasions, good-humored George Ohsawa
would introduce me to guests, "Look at that girl. She came
from the deep Izumo mountains. We call her Masakari because she once brought an axe into the tatami room."

Once I made a poem about a garden of scallions. This
caused him to introduce me as Hiding in the Scallion Garden
Axe. Explaining this nickname to newcomers, he would make
a pun on *uta* which meant poem and *nuta* which meant miso
dressing.

A lifelong advocate of reviving the beautiful Japanese
language, George always said that a person who could not
write poems was not a true person. He himself wrote a lot of
poems. Several years later, he and Lima set off on a voyage to
India. The ship they were traveling on, *Sadhana*, mysteriously
lost its compass bearings while passing through the Straits of
Molucca. Meditating on this strange occurrence, George realized it was on account of encountering countless spirits of
soldiers who had died during World War II. He and Lima

vowed to fast for the day. After composing some beautiful verses for the wandering souls and rededicating his life for peace, the ship started functioning normally again.

One day, in the main house, Alcan Yamaguchi slapped me for impudent behavior toward the boys in the school. He said that my emotions were not like a girl's. There was a big debate that night. Is Alcan or Axe right? Only Parfait spoke up in my behalf. George Ohsawa just listened, laughing, with no comment.

Another time, I don't remember why, a fifteen-year-old boy from a nearby reformatory came to dinner. George Ohsawa was very happy and gave him the name Rocky. He referred to him affectionately many times during his lectures. Rocky's appearance was a little insolent and precocious, and he gave the feeling of being more of an adult than a child. Two or three days passed. When pocket money started disappearing at the M.I., our suspicions turned to Rocky. We went to find him but he had already disappeared. George Ohsawa was very sad and unhappy. He scolded us bitterly, "Ten to fifteen of you live together with Rocky. But nobody could reach his heart." He stopped the morning lecture, and everyone went out to find him. With two or three friends, I searched in the back of a nearby field where wheat was growing. Others went to the train station. Three stops from Hiyoshi, Rocky was located in a candy store. He came back, and everyone was very nice to him. But soon he ran away again. This happened several times, and finally he went away for good.

Gradually I began to understand George Ohsawa's teachings. I eagerly looked forward to his lectures, especially on peaceful Sunday mornings in spring and on quiet rainy evenings. His basic message was always freedom. Many times he said, "You are free to do anything in this world. You don't need to observe human laws and boundaries. They are unnatural. You don't need to be afraid of anything. Your decisions and actions are entirely up to you. Even if you rob a bank or injure people, do not worry about the law of punishment. If you kill one person, you may be called a murderer and go to prison. But if you kill one hundred people, you are a war hero. In one minute we are able to kill millions of people today. The inventors of the atomic bomb received the Nobel Prize for their efforts. In the name of modern medicine, see how many people are killed day by day. Too many to count. Are the Nobel Prize winners helping humanity or not? They are not really dedicated to human happiness, truth, and justice in this world. There is nothing like absolute justice or absolute goodness in this life. You have to do what you like, carry out your own dream."

Listening to his words reverberating intensely and cheerfully we felt a tremendous release. We felt our hearts were as one, and we could do anything. Suddenly all of us felt as if we were emboldened, completely free, and our ways of life were opened forever.

"But there is one law we must not break for a free and happy life," he concluded as his lectures reached a climax. "That is the Order of the Universe, the law of nature. It is the only condition. In Far Eastern philosophy it is said, 'Heaven's net is very big and roughly woven. But you cannot cheat and pass through.' Heaven's vengeance is slow but sure. Even if we can avoid and violate the laws in this world, we can never hide and escape from the Order of the Universe. Where there is a cause, there is an effect. If we break the laws of nature, we immediately get sick, become unhappy, and die."

Quoting Samuel Butler's *Erewhon*, he would say that sick people should be sent to jail and criminals should be sent to the hospital. In astonishment, we realized how difficult and severe the Order of the Universe was compared with the ease of breaking human laws.

Around that time, a famous statesman, Toshio Tamura, came to stay at the M.I. He was a consultant to Prime Minister Ikeda and Minister of Education in Manchuria during the war. When at Hiyoshi, he stayed in room number 6, nicknamed the Sixth Heaven, next to George Ohsawa's room number 7, the Seventh Heaven. His friendship with Ohsawa went back to the war. Convinced of Japan's imminent defeat,

Ohsawa left on a one-man peace mission to Moscow to get
Soviet Premier Joseph Stalin to negotiate an end to hostilities
between Japan and the United States. Ohsawa's route took
him through Manchuria, where in the 50 degree below zero
temperatures of winter he hoped to ride on horseback through
enemy lines to Siberia and catch the Trans-Siberian railroad
to the Russian capital. In the Manchurian capital, Ohsawa was
promptly caught by the Japanese military and ordered before
a firing squad. But before he could be shot, Mr. Tamura, who
had read and respected his translation of Alexis Carrel's book,
secured his release. He returned to Japan to plot other ways
to bring the fighting to an end.

George Ohsawa's strong, violent type of instruction may
have grown out of experiences such as this. In lectures he
would often say, "In wartime, in the field of battle, if you
don't report or communicate well, great trouble will result.
You may lose one thousand people because of miscommunication. Prompt and efficient reporting and clear expression are
essential. You must know that."

Mr. Tamura, whose P.U. name was Tovarisch (Russian
for Comrade) helped George Ohsawa with the translation of
a new book recently published in America, *The Meeting of
East and West*. George felt that the author, F. M. C. Northrup
a philosophy teacher at Yale, understood the Unique Principle
and enthusiastically prepared to bring it before the Japanese
reading public. Tovarisch sometimes spoke at lectures. He
talked smilingly about the pleasure of hunger. "When someone becomes angry, tired, or weak, that shows poor health.
When someone becomes very happy, it is because inside they
are very hungry. The hungrier they are, the happier they
become. That's real health." To emphasize his point, he would
put his hands in the belt around his waist and show how skinny
he had grown since coming to the M.I.

Like many newcomers, Tovarisch was surprised at the
plainness and faint-heartedness of the students at Maison
Ignoramus. "Why don't you have more elite students?" he
once asked.

"We have a test in this school," George Ohsawa replied, "H.H.T., the Health and Happiness Test. This test doesn't require a consultant or fortune-teller to detect your life's direction. Here you determine your own destiny. It must be done in just forty minutes. There are many questions to fill out, and then you grade yourself. The difference between this test and others is that someone with the lowest marks has more qualifications. You can enter any time, any day. When you find out how ignorant you really are, then you graduate."

The test he referred to was a simple question and answer test. "Do you have a strong appetite?" "How many hours do you sleep?" "Is your energy always up?" So many points were given for each reply. We marked the answers to the questions while looking at a clock.

"The students here are not so smart, not so beautiful, and most of them are poor," Ohsawa continued in reply to Tovarisch's question. "They are like frogs living under the sand in a deep well who know nothing of the world. To change them and enable them to see a larger, brighter, healthier world is my greatest happiness."

In the autumn, about eight or nine months after I came to Hiyoshi, George Ohsawa took me aside. He gave me the name Aveline. He said that he had made it up from "Ave Maria," referring to Mary the mother of Jesus, and "line," a common suffix as in "Caroline" or "Angeline." I was deeply moved at being given a saint's name and felt I did not deserve it. But overwhelmed with his confidence in me, I changed my name from Asta to Aveline and have used it every day since. Perhaps he chose it because of my Christian heritage. After studying yin and yang with him, my own understanding of the Bible and Jesus's teachings of love and compassion greatly increased.

From the early hours of the morning till late at night, George Ohsawa was constantly active—writing, reading, carrying on a worldwide correspondence, cleaning, lecturing, dreaming of the new world to come. He had a mountain of ideas to tell us. But we were dumb and didn't understand

114

anything. Such poor girls and boys, our strongest desire was for food. Yet he continued teaching us patiently day after day. Only when we didn't answer right away would he rebuke us like a stern father, "Oh, you're dead."

George Ohsawa was a fascinating combination of personalities. Sometimes he was a saint, sometimes a dandy, sometimes an old farmer, sometimes a gangster. He assumed many characters and had an endless appetite for life. Because of his own strong character, he tended to repel as many people as he attracted such as table-pounding Mr. Nagata who studied for a while and never came back. Nor did he appeal very much to people his own age who were pursuing official careers or to scholars, who thought they had a monopoly on knowledge. But he appealed to the common people, the widowed and orphaned, the sick and the fearful—the salt of the earth.

My abiding memories are of his talking about the Unique Principle, smoking a pipe, and calling on Pascal, Augustine, and other famous Western thinkers after whom he had named his students and on whom he counted to change the world. He was constantly in motion, pushing, prodding, criticizing, exhorting. Yet inside I could detect a calm, warm heart. Strange and fun, stimulating and deep, that was life at Maison Ignoramus.

6: The Samurai of Shinjuku Station

"My dear Asta, we don't know when we can meet, but I cannot forget your kind spirit. This is very strongly felt and carved like a sculpture in my heart, deeper than the Olympian gods carved in the Parthenon. Our real purpose is to appreciate life in all its wonder and beauty. Let's together follow in Jesus's footsteps and observe George Ohsawa's patient, quiet, and deep teachings."—Michio Kushi, first letter to Aveline

GEORGE OHSAWA always lectured with a blackboard behind him. In the lefthand corner, he kept the names of several students. On top was the name of Michio Kushi. Many times at the end of his talks, he would say, "Please follow Michio's step." Michio had come to Hiyoshi to study with George Ohsawa while completing his graduate studies in the international political science department of Tokyo University. He was a member of the United World Federalists and deeply committed to the cause of world government and world peace. With the help of Norman Cousins, Michio became the first student of George Ohsawa's to go to America. There had been a big farewell party for him at Maison Ignoramus in November, about three months before my arrival. Attired in a tuxedo, silk top hat, and carrying a cane, a jaunty George Ohsawa saw him off on the *General Golden*, an ocean liner bound for the West Coast.

One beautiful April morning, after breakfast George Ohsawa appeared for the morning lecture. He was so happy that he was almost dancing and jumping for joy. "We just received a letter from Michio," he said waving an envelope with foreign stamps. Since leaving Japan, Michio hadn't sent any news, and everyone was very curious about how he was faring. With great emotion, George Ohsawa read the letter in a deep, clear voice as we breathlessly listened. It opened with the greeting, "Dear Everyone, My Friends," and described the small dark apartment he lived in by the Hudson River in New York City. He told about finding a lamp to read by during the day. In Japan we couldn't imagine needing lamps in daytime and thought the shoji screens in America must be very strange not to let in sufficient light.

Later that day, in the editorial offices where I was helping out, George Ohsawa asked me to copy out Michio's letter for the printer. He wanted to publish it in the World Government newspaper, and it had to be transcribed on special graph paper with one ideograph to a box for the typesetter. I was very pleased to be asked because it was such a beautiful letter. Also, Michio's handwriting was very poetic. Composed in normal size characters and written on ordinary paper, it was a welcome change from the usual scraps of his own dashed off jottings that George Ohsawa gave me to decipher.

That night I copied out the letter, and it was so moving I wept. I cried many times while reading poetry and literature. Right after the war, a beautiful novel, *Harp of Burma*, came out. I cried so loudly Mother came to check and found me teary-eyed, the book open on my lap. Once again, tears flowed, touching my heart, as I copied out Michio's writing. Someday, somewhere, I thought to myself, I'd like to meet him. I had fallen in love with Michio through his letter.

George Ohsawa asked everyone to reply to Michio, and I sent the first letter, enclosing some of my poems.

I asked Darbin what Michio looked like. She said he had never lived at the dorm but came and went by train from his campus in Tokyo. She remembered he was a nice person but recalled he had holes in his socks. I also learned that Michio was born in Wakayama province, the same region where George Ohsawa came from, and that both his parents were teachers. George Ohsawa said that Michio inherited his mother's strong constitution but while growing up developed a more yin, tubercular condition. But because he didn't eat much sugar, he survived.

Street sales of the World Government newspaper were the M.I.'s chief source of income. Circulars for the monthly paper proclaimed that it was "edited, published, and sold for the last three years in the ruined streets of Japan under the rage of waves of suicides, crimes, and inflation after the war by the self-supporting boys and girls of the Student World Government Association." In lectures, George Ohsawa was always telling us to be self-reliant. "Don't become a slave by taking a salary. Salaries are like chains. When I see a schoolteacher or office worker, I can hear the sound of their chains dragging behind them. Be your own master. Create your own job."

I decided to try my hand at selling newspapers. Unlike Mitsuko, the champion insurance saleswoman, I had no experience in sales. My only previous occasion asking people for money was very embarrassing. In our family, the children helped Father by going around to farms and collecting cash for credit slips before the New Year. It was the part of the holiday season I dreaded. I was still shy and apprehensive about asking people for money. But I was very proud to carry newspapers containing Michio Kushi's beautiful article.

The M.I. news vendors usually worked in small groups or pairs. I set off with Juste, the young teenager. Some parts of Tokyo were totally destroyed. In the once fashionable Ginza we often sat down in a bombed-out field and ate rice balls for lunch. One day I sold about thirty copies very easily. I just walked down Kanda, a famous street, and surprised people strolling by.

The greatest concentration of people was at the train stations. Tokyo Station, the hub of the city's busy rail network, had been heavily damaged during the war. The back side was demolished, with construction crews laying new track and making other repairs behind a forest of plywood fences. In the front of the station, some young people were hawking *Akahata* ("Red Flag"), the communist newspaper. Rather than compete with them, I decided to sell inside the terminal where people were waiting for trains or sitting on benches. At first I approached people one by one, patiently explaining world government and the connection between health and diet, hoping to convince them to buy. I had not spoken with many persons before a girl in a station uniform came by and told me I couldn't sell in the terminal. I left.

After that, I decided to go directly up to the train platforms. In Tokyo there is a round circuit line. The purchase of a single ticket allowed you to ride all day, so long as you didn't leave the elevated station area. I soon discovered which sections of the city were receptive to news of world government activities and which were not. The best was Waseda University. There the students were keenly interested, and I had many earnest conversations on world peace. Tokyo University, Michio's alma mater, was also very good. Keio University was harder. The students came from richer families and appeared less interested in new ideas. The least interested were those from Gakushū-in, the college for members of the Imperial family and nobility. They struck me as being weak and not at all serious. In this way, I could see the school spirit simply by selling newspapers.

Generally, I left the M.I. with my papers about noon and returned by 5 P.M. for dinner and the evening lecture. I tried to go out with some of the other girls. But they were a little weak and couldn't keep up with me. The boys and I left the dormitory with big bundles of two to three hundred papers and put most of them in a storage locker in Shibuya Station on the circle line. We would take a small amount, sell them, and come back for more. Some of my articles started to appear in the World Government newspaper, further boosting my self-confidence.

Selling newspapers in the stations was not permitted. The guards often caught me and marched me to the station office where they had me write out a statement, "I'm sorry I came to sell newspapers. This is illegal. I won't do it any more." I signed the statement but was back on the platforms with my

newspapers the next day. This happened again and again.
One day, in Shinjuku Station, my favorite spot, I was ap-
prehended and conducted to an office in a high building by
the station. An official asked me to sit down.

"Why are you coming here so often?" he asked producing
a stack of about thirty statements I had signed. "You promised not to come back. Still you came again today. Your
handwriting is so beautiful. What is the matter?"

"I really wish no more war," I replied. "Don't you think
so?"

"Yes, of course," he answered.

"That's why I come here, so there should be no more world
war."

He relaxed. We conversed about world peace and I introduced to him George Ohsawa's activities. No conclusion was
reached. I left and continued my selling. The station personnel
continued to detain me. But after that they were more respectful, "We understand what you are doing. Please understand
this is our job."

As the weeks and months passed, I found that selling newspapers was the best training I had ever had. I began to understand the essence of macrobiotics. Even the number of sales
depended on my day-to-day physical and mental condition.
I started to know ahead of time who would buy and who
wouldn't just by observing people sitting or standing at the
station.

For example, to a middle-aged man I might say:

"If you read the World Government newspaper, you will
become younger."

"That's impossible," he'd reply.

"Yes, it can be," I'd say.

"You are young," he would come back. "That's why you
are a dreamer."

"You are old, that's why you give up," I'd respond.

"Ha, ha, ha. You say funny things. I can't defeat or fight
with you. Ha, ha, ha. I will take one."

Another time, I had conversations that went like this:

"Read *World Government*. If you read, you will become happy or fortunate."

—"Something funny is written here."

"Yes, of course, it's all funny things."

—"We don't need that."

"If you read, it really helps you. Suppose you take this train. Trouble may develop. It may turn upside down or end up in the water just like that accident several days ago."

—"Don't say such bad things."

"That's all right. Even so, at those times you will know how to escape. Such things are written here."

—"You say good things."

"Take one."

—"Oh, you made me buy!"

Sometimes I would mention a famous person who was active in world government activities.

"Please read about the World Government movement. It is something like what Professor Einstein is doing."

—"Einstein? I don't care what Einstein is doing."

"What's the meaning of 'don't care'?"

—"I forget already what Einstein did."

"That's OK, you can forget. But if you really want peace, you can't forget this."

—"I think I'll take one. Thank you very much."

One day George Ohsawa went out of town for a seminar. For a whole week I wouldn't have to worry about missing his lectures. I decided to sell from early morning to late at night, eating only brown rice, the famous number 7 diet he later popularized. My sales soared. I found that people were attracted to me even if I didn't approach them. I discovered that the station guards no longer caught me. I became transparent.

I found that the less I spoke, the more papers I could sell. Finally, I reached the point where I would just bow once when the passengers got off the train and extend the World Government publication to them. Without thinking, they would put their hands in their pocket and hand me the money. I felt just like a samurai. Except instead of killing people with a sword, I was giving out papers on all sides—left, right, front, and back—that offered them new life. In a few minutes, my bundle would be all gone.

Once, during the week, I ate some leftover *udon* noodles. That day my sales dropped by half. On just brown rice, my body felt very light. I set a new sales record, 350 papers a day. The other students at M.I. marveled and said I had the same activity level as George Ohsawa. It was a wonderful feeling. Taking the train back at night was like going to heaven. One day, I decided to walk back to the dormitory and got off at the station before Hiyoshi. A sudden downpour came, and I walked back in the rain by myself, thoroughly soaked, singing as I went. That was the essence of my education with George Ohsawa. We change according to what we eat and our day-to-day condition. Our health and happiness are entirely up to ourselves.

One day in late spring, George Ohsawa sent me to the post office with a registered letter. I came back and forgot to give him the receipt. He asked me where it was. I went to look but couldn't find it. Giving up, I went to lunch. Later, Lima came to the table and said, "Before you located the receipt, you are eating. Papa is very angry. You must find it." I looked everywhere but the paper couldn't be found.

The most severe form of punishment at the dormitory was exile. The student would be told, "You can no longer stay here. It is time for you to go." Many times I saw this happen. Lima would deliver the message from the Seventh Heaven.

My punishment was less severe. She told me I could no longer attend lectures but must go out and sell newspapers the whole day. For a couple of days I obeyed, but I could not stand to sell any more. My mind was still on the lectures, which were the most joyful and happiest part of the day. George Ohsawa's talks were the heart and essence of life at the M.I. and the reason I came to stay. I decided to listen secretly to George Ohsawa speak from the next room. Japanese homes have thin paper walls, and it is easy to hear what's being said on the other side. I hid in the next room during the lectures. In the mornings, I found that while listening I could even take advantage of not being seen to fold all my newspapers for the day.

After awhile, knowing full well that I was listening in, George Ohsawa would tell students in the back of the room to slide the door open a little to let some air in. It became just like a game between us for several months. Finally, one day during a monthly birthday party, Lima notified me that the ban had been lifted.

But even parties were not exempt from Papa's scorn. On another occasion, he brought some cake and other party food to the M.I. and left it out on the table for the students to enjoy. He was always saying you could eat anything you wanted if you were truly healthy and understood the Unique Principle. Most of the boys and girls happily ate it. One other student and myself didn't touch it. Later, we found out that the cake contained sugar and that he was testing our judgment and will power. Chiding everyone who had eaten the cake, George Ohsawa said we should all automatically have sensed that it had sugar. None of us was strong or free enough to handle sugar. "Even when you know medicine, you shouldn't fool around with poison," he warned.

Michio's second letter arrived during the summer. It was long, about twenty pages. It began with a commentary on life in America. He used the Unique Principle to explain the paradox of the world's mightiest nation suffering postwar economic and political problems. Then to each of the students who had written him, he offered personal comments, including a brief note to me.

To Asta, my friend whom I have not seen,
    Your letter gladdens my heart and infuses it with a surprising fire. I think this comes from your constitution,

personality, and aesthetic sensibility. Here it is often very busy and tense. My smile has a tendency to fade, but your letter has brought it back. I think that love appears in the simplest expression of words and feelings.

Many times people in present-day society laugh at or criticize our thoughts and movement. Such difficulties may occur from time to time, but we should not lose our smiles and always keep loving those who abuse us. I'm sure your beautiful heart will think kindly and shed a tear for us over here. To listen to your words is like facing the morning sun, which brightens everyone's dreams and wishes with its radiance. I hope if everything goes well, I can send you my poor poems. Your beautiful words go deeply into my heart.

My dear Asta, we don't know when we can meet, but I cannot forget your kind spirit. This is very strongly felt and carved like a sculpture in my heart, deeper than the Olympian gods carved in the Parthenon. Our real purpose is to appreciate life in all its wonder and beauty. Let's together follow in Jesus's footsteps and observe George Ohsawa's patient, quiet, and deep teachings.

My dear friend, Asta, I think that many, many friends would be pleased to follow your beautiful spirit when they come to know you. You inspire me deeply.

Though Michio wrote to many of the girls, I noted that his reply to me was the most romantic.

Because of his quixotic activites during the war, George Ohsawa was still on a list of people barred from leaving Japan. Although he could not yet travel, it was his dream to send twelve disciples abroad to spread macrobiotics. He counted Michio as his number 1 ambassador for world government. Several boys, including Pascal, Augustine, and Gabon, had gone to France, where George Ohsawa still had many contacts. André Shimizu, a young man from Hamamatsu, and a Christian minister from Hokkaido left for the United States. Mr. Shinohara went to Chicago, and Roman Sato went to

Los Angeles. In some cases, their visits were brief and they returned home.

One of George Ohsawa's favorite pastimes was writing letters, manifestos, and appeals to world leaders explaining his teachings and asking for their support. He eagerly awaited their replies each month but rarely got a response. One of the few who did answer personally was Dr. Albert Schweitzer in Africa. Because of his commitment to world government, George Ohsawa received invitations to send representatives to world peace congresses. As the Cold War between America and Russia heated up, Prime Minister Nehru of India, Thomas Mann, Upton Sinclair, Norman Cousins, and other prominent World Federalists sponsored assemblies for people from around the world to meet and discuss ways to avert an atomic arms race and create a new international order. The Student World Government Association in Hiyoshi was one of the few world government centers in Japan.

It was very difficult to leave Japan at that time. Everyone was very poor, and on the international exchange Japanese yen were worthless. For several months, I helped promote attendance at these conferences and helped George Ohsawa look for suitable representatives from universities and civic groups who might be in a position to represent us. But most people were more interested in travel for its own sake than for world government. Gradually, I realized that I would make the best delegate. I started to dream of traveling. In the January issue of *Le Compas*, George Ohsawa's small monthly magazine, I listed going to a world peace congress as one of my top ten accomplishments or resolutions of the year. I listed it just ahead of discovering Michio's existence and losing my fear of sickness.

About that time, word came of a world federalist assembly in Paris. One morning, I wrote a poem about spreading our vision of the world.

Let's Go

Let's go!
Our preparation is finished.
There is no need to carry two cloaks.
The soft, beautiful grass and the trees and buds are all
     opened, full of green.
The May rain is melting away the cold of winter.
Let's go!
When golden sunshine bursts forth
Let's tie our shoestrings
And set out!

Earlier that morning, George Ohsawa decided to give me
permission to travel abroad. I held the record for sales of the
World Government newspaper, and he thought I would make
a good ambassador for the Unique Principle. He hadn't told
me yet when I gave him the poem. Afterwards, everyone
marveled and said I must have ESP.

I couldn't believe my good fortune. My happy mood was
expressed in another poem that went like this:

Wonder

I wonder.
Sometimes I wonder
Why tall, skinny George Ohsawa wears Chinese-style
     dress.
We try to catch the May rain in Shinjuku
And run with Mama (Lima).
I wonder.
I really wonder,
Can I go to U.S.?
Farewell, I'm going to America
and will start to work for the whole world.
I hope everyone will come together with me.
I wonder.

I wonder what is the origin of wonder.
Please come.

The first problem was arranging my travel documents. To
get to France, I had to take a boat to the West Coast, cross
America by bus or train, and then take another boat to Europe.
To get an American transit visa, I needed a French visa. To
get a French visa, I had to have financial guarantees.

One of the M.I. students knew a Chinese merchant, Mr.
Wang, who ran a successful business in the South Pacific. He
supported the goal of world government. I went to see him
at his home in Tokyo and asked for a letter of guarantee. He
had an account with the Chase Manhattan Bank, but since he
didn't know me was afraid to be my sponsor. Finally he
signed the letter. Abe typed it up for me, along with an embel-
lished account of my reasons for traveling and itinerary. I
presented it at the French Embassy but was still turned down.

Undaunted, I kept returning to the French Embassy every
day in hope that they would change their mind. One day, I
arrived at lunchtime and all the regular French clerks had
stepped out. One old Japanese officer was behind the desk.
I handed him my papers. With trembling hands and perspiration dripping from his brow, he quickly stamped my passport. Later, we invited him to visit the Maison Ignoramus and
explained our cause. He said he was convinced by my sincere
heart to give me the visa and knew destiny had brought us
together. After getting the French visa, I went to the American Embassy and received a one-month travel visa. The old
man's superiors soon found out that I had been granted a
stamp and cancelled my French visa. But by then, I had permission to visit America and no longer really cared whether
I reached Paris or not.

Having a passport and foreign visa also helped me sell
newspapers and promote macrobiotics. Among ourselves, we
called our adventures fishing expeditions. One of the biggest
catches I reeled in for the M.I. was a young man subsequently
known as Balzac. I fished him from Shinjuku Station. He was

working for the U.S. Army photographing technical maps. The Korean war had just started.

"It was snowing, and I thought Aveline a strange and interesting girl standing on the platform with her newspapers," he recalled many years later. "I thought I would tease her and struck up a conversation." He remembered what followed.

"Please read about world government," I said handing him a newspaper.

"World government is a dream in a dream," he scoffed.

"I may not look so fancy, but I'm going to New York," I replied.

Balzac was shocked. "After the war," he recalled, "everyone wanted to travel to a foreign country. But no one could go. It was like living in a cave. Even government ministers had difficulty making arrangements to go to America. It was inconceivable this young girl had a visa."

"I don't believe you," he exclaimed. "Show me."

"Will you believe it now?" I said, taking out my passport.

"I wanted a visa too," Balzac reminisced. "I promised her I would attend a lecture and came to Hiyoshi the next week. George Ohsawa was most impressive. He emphasized *non credo*, think for yourself. That was the beginning of my involvement."

Balzac remained active in the movement for several years, visiting macrobiotic friends in Europe. Later he went on to set up a successful company in Tokyo making strobe lights.

I also fished a big newspaper writer for the *Yomiuri Shimbun*, whom I brought to George Ohsawa. My friend, Aida, who later accompanied me many times, snagged Tomio Kikuchi. After studying in Hiyoshi, he went to Brazil and has been one of the main macrobiotic teachers in Latin America over the last three decades.

Mr. Kikuchi's future wife, another girl Ohsawa named Bernadette, also studied at the M.I. and succeeded me as the record holder. In later years, Lima liked to tell how the girls supported the boys at Hiyoshi. "We gave North America to Aveline and South America to Bernadette because they sold so many World Government newspapers. Their husbands just followed behind. The girls' spirit put our minds at ease about the future of macrobiotics in the West."

Once my visa was obtained, the next problem was getting a ticket. I had no money. George Ohsawa introduced me to Oritaro Shimizu, who had helped finance the foreign travel of his son, André, a student at the M.I. I went to see Mr. Shimizu at his home in Hamamatsu, a big city between Tokyo and Kyoto. He owned several silk-weaving factories that had been destroyed in the bombing and was now farming in the countryside. A calm, energetic man, with bright, smiling eyes and large, well-formed ears, Mr. Shimizu listened sympathetically to my appeal. His philosophy of life was that:

Man should be like the heart of the sun.
Woman should be like the heart of a flower.

Unperturbed by the loss of his own home, factories, and land in the war, he promised to help. "We are like dandelions blown in the wind," he explained. "Destiny decides for us when it is time to move." Although he had no cash himself, he borrowed fifty thousand yen—a small fortune—from neighboring rice farmers. Mr. Shimizu's generosity enabled me to buy my tickets.

Before leaving on my trip, I went home to visit my family. I returned with a suitcase full of World Government newspapers and copies of George Ohsawa's book about Jack and Yo-Yo's adventures in the land of Erewhon. My mother, sisters, and brothers were glad to see me. Although they still didn't understand macrobiotics, they could see that I was in excellent spirits. I also visited my college teacher, Mr. Tanaka in Shiga, a lakeside resort near Kyoto. It was the first time we had seen each other since my sickness when he found me "very weak and pitifully skinny" in bed. He was glad to see me and observed that "a peaceful and new Miss Yokoyama was born, who was as free as before, full of passion, but not too extraordinary." I shared some unpolished rice balls I brought with him. He noticed they were a little moldy.

I assured him they were still nutritious.

Mr. Tanaka was very interested in my studies. He readily saw the relation between Ninomiya's teachings and macro-biotics. Later he met George Ohsawa and thanked him for helping me. Mr. Tanaka told him he wasn't surprised I went to America. He also went to see Mother in Yokota and put flowers on Father's grave.

I also visited Ken-chan, my childhood friend, who was living near Kyoto. He had completed his veterinary studies and was working in a town near the Old Capital. I presented him with macrobiotic literature, but he was still very active in church affairs and not so interested in this approach.

Back in Tokyo, I completed preparations for my journey. I said goodbye to friends I had made over the last year and a half, including one of the guards at Shinjuku Station. "I'm sorry I disturbed you so much," I said. "I won't come any more from tomorrow." He was surprised and envious. "Some-day we shall see you again," he smiled, waving back.

My fellow students at the M.I. gave me a farewell party. I invited a man whom I met sketching in a corner of the plat-form at Shinjuku Station to come. His name was Mr. Ono and at the party he made a drawing of me.

The next morning in Hiyoshi, I went to say goodbye to George Ohsawa. "Everything is prepared. What shall I do?"

"Do you have any last questions?" he replied.

"Is it all right to drink milk?" I asked. The question came to me out of the blue. I had never seen cheese and most dairy products before but knew they were eaten every day in the United States.

"No, you don't need," he said emphatically and went back into his room.

Several friends accompanied me to Tokyo Station, and we exchanged goodbyes on the platform.

Alcan Yamaguchi, the editor of the World Government newspaper, later published an article about my departure. My trip, the first by a girl at the M.I., was known as Women's Caravan number 1. The article ran under that headline:

Miss Aveline Yokoyama, a salesgirl for this newspaper, is going to leave for the United States. She first plans to visit Michio Kushi in New York and help with his World Government activities. From there she will go to Paris and meet other caravan members in Geneva. Later, George Ohsawa will attend. He plans to accompany Men' Caravan number 4 or number 5 and will join friends together in Europe. Outside of Paris, he will establish an Academy of Freedom. Aveline Yokoyama will study there with all the other caravan members. That is her schedule. . . .

Last February, she left her home region of Shimane Prefecture. Her great dream and passion was to meet George Ohsawa. She traveled alone to Tokyo to the M.I. Under his guidance, she has been pursuing world government activities for the last year and five months. Rain, sun, or snow, she has sold the World Government newspaper continually without hesitation.

For readers of this newspaper, you may have seen her on the platform of Shinjuku Station. To understand her devotion, just recall back to last October 18. On his birthday, George Ohsawa announced the gathering of the first People's World Congress in Europe. He asked for volunteers to attend. Aveline was the first one to open her mouth. Everyone was surprised and shocked. In December, we sent four men to Europe. Aveline put more and more effort into selling newspapers. Sometimes the guards and police caught her and forced her to sign many confessions. Many times on the station platform, guards and staff of the station asked her to leave. *World Government* became famous thanks to Miss Yokoyama. Many people became friendly with her. Sometimes she stayed out till midnight. One day she sold more than 300 copies. Then she set a new record with 350 newspapers. It is very difficult ordinarily to sell 100 papers a day. She made the impossible possible. George Ohsawa told her

that she had graduated. She passed the test of freedom.
She was now a free person.

George Ohsawa realized this and authorized her to go.
Aveline started applying for a passport and visa. She
started on June 18. Day and night, Abe Nakamura typed
for her, and Mr. Shimizu and several other people gave
her financial support. In one week she completed her arrangements to travel. This is really a miracle. On June
26, she left Tokyo in the evening. . . . She was very emotional and cried. Tears streamed down the cheeks of
everyone else too. Many guards and staff at Tokyo
Station came to say goodbye.

We cannot forget her tremendous progress. The year
before she came, she was very sick. After surviving this
life-or-death illness, she came to Tokyo. Every day until
late at night, she sold newspapers and set the record.
Now on her departure for America, she is very happy and
healthy. She realized that the secret of macrobiotics is
natural medicine. You shouldn't miss it either.

When she came in February, after her sickness, her
face was very red. It looked just like the *kaki* fruit which
grows in her home country or the face of a monkey.
She also had a deep line on her forehead. Biologically,
these things have meaning. Now that face is completely
changed. She looks younger and more natural. The line
has disappeared too. Also her personality has changed.
She was very proud, tight, and narrow. She was more
like a boy, very defensive. She changed. Her tightness
softened, more like a lady's. She started to cry. She
changed physically and spiritually. The credit goes to
George Ohsawa who has been teaching the Unique Principle and the Order of the Universe for forty years. This
is an example of macrobiotics. This is the basis of world
government. The biological revolution of humanity is the
essence of world government. By changing her condition,
she can change the world. For millions of years of human

history, no one has explained this well until now. The world is full of fighting, war, and suffering. Aveline Yokoyama is traveling for peace and freedom. She will spread light wherever she goes. She is Women's Caravan number 1.

Along with this article, the students published my last poem

Please Distribute

Please distribute *World Government*.
Run around and shout, "World Government, World
  Government."
To sell *World Government* is the highest task in human
  life.
Fighting and confusion is spreading in society.
The light is going out.
Please restore it.
Light the lost light of humanity's eternal dream.
Go forth and distribute *World Government*.
One by one, each person's life can be lit.
Their candleholders may already be worn and tired.
Even those of old men and ladies can be rekindled.
And those of young men who are floating through life
Can become beautiful, transparent, and strong again.
Give up and leave everything else behind.
Let's relight humanity's dying flame.
Run, run around to sell *World Government*
Even if you are punished and put in jail,
Do this for the sake of our eternal dream.

After saying goodbye to my fellow students, I took the train to Kobe, Japan's main port, in the Osaka-Kyoto area. I stayed at a friend's house. It was the first week in July and the weather was hot and sultry. Mother came to see me off. I carried my boat ticket and a Greyhound Bus ticket from San Francisco to New York but no money. My last few yen were spent on some straw sandals.

Garry Davis's story in a French magazine and the *New York Times* that spring had made a deep impression on us. The young ex-bomber pilot had renounced his American nationality in Paris and declared himself a world citizen. For the last several years, he had traveled around the world without any money or passport challenging arbitrary laws and boundaries. He had been jailed countless times but somehow always managed to keep his sense of humor and get by. George Ohsawa really admired Garry's spirit and adventures and told us to try it for ourselves. Although I was about the same age as Garry, I felt Mr. Ohsawa was a little worried about sending a young Japanese girl to America without a penny.

From my side, I was never afraid and counted on the spirit of love and truth after which I was named to see me through. Shortly before I left, I received a letter from Michio saying that my verse had "stopped his heart from beating" and comparing my words to "the strings of a beautiful instrument." The poem he enclosed made reference to the unhappy life of the poor people he observed in Manhattan.

The stars are spiralling,
And Spring has come again.
The white clouds stream overhead
As I start to sing
Of the decaying city around me.
My heart is unsettled.
Tears flow but I do not wipe them away.
My voice trembles
At the sadness and misery I see.
I sing a deep, melancholy song.

On July 6, I bid farewell to Mother, and she gave me some rice balls for the long journey. The steamer weighed anchor, passing the picturesque coastline of Wakayama province where Michio was born. I was anxious to see in person the tender spirit this beautiful country of steep mountains, high waterfalls, delicate orange blossoms, and ancient shrines had produced. Through deep waves, the ship continued to Nagoya, its last cargo stop. From there, the vessel rounded the snowy canopy of Mt. Fuji and the lush Izu peninsula and made for the open sea. I composed many poems as the land of my birth vanished from sight and the land of my dreams drew closer.

7: Journey Across the Eastern Sea

"From Michio, I am learning to feel a great yearning
for humanity. He feels that the human race is sinking
down in a deep pond without a bottom. He hopes to
stop it with World Government. He talks passionately about a new world order and really devotes all
his energies to this cause."—Aveline, Letter to friends
at the M.I.

OUT OF KOBE, the beautiful, long white Norweigan
steamship *Colona* carried seven passengers enroute to
San Francisco besides its cargo and crew. I shared a
cabin with a Russian lady named Anna. Neither of us spoke the
other's language. There was a New York businessman on the
voyage, but my English was not good enough to communicate
with him either. My main travel companion was an American
lady, the principal of a Catholic girls' school in Tokyo, who
knew some Japanese. She had served as tutor to the Crown
Prince. It was the middle of July, the time of the mid-summer
Bon festival, and on deck I danced one evening by moonlight.

We ate together at one table with the captain and crew
in a galley belowdecks. The only thing I could eat was Norweigan flatbread, made of rye and wheat. Before I left,
Darbin made me some roasted rice which fluffed up like rice
crispies but was chewy, and I ate a little of that each day in
my cabin.

To make some pocket money, I offered to wash clothing
for the crew. But one of the sailors came to hug me, and I
decided to stop. Except for this incident, two weeks of un-

broken horizons, salt spray, and thin, dry wafers passed peacefully. The evening before reaching the West Coast, the teacher
insisted I eat some vegetables at dinner. I had been avoiding
vegetables because I knew they were cooked in beef stock.
But to please her, I tried some boiled carrots, green peas, and
broccoli. That night, for the first time since becoming macrobiotic over a year and a half earlier, I had bad dreams. A wild
dog chased me to the top of a hill from which I tried to escape.
I had never experienced such a nightmare before and woke
up perspiring all over.

It was a beautiful sunny day. Strong waves followed in our
wake as the ship glided under the Golden Gate Bridge into
San Francisco Harbor. I had a terrible headache and suddenly
remembered the food I had eaten the previous night. I understood clearly the cause of my discomfort and saw that happiness and unhappiness were entirely up to me. George Ohsawa
had taught us that food shapes consciousness and behavior.
But this was the first time I really experienced the effects of
poor quality food after eating well for a long time and im-
proving my condition. As I stepped onto American soil, it was
a great realization.

At customs, my Russian cabin mate was held up because she
was coughing. Immigration officials suspected she had tuberculosis. I thought I might be detained but was waved right
through. The steamship company gave me an $8 tax refund
on my ticket, so I now had some money in my pocket. A young
Japanese-American woman met me at the pier. She was the
daughter of a Seventh Day Adventist minister who George
Ohsawa had arranged to meet me. They had also befriended
Michio on his arrival in America two years before. The girl
led me to a car and, to my surprise, took the wheel herself.
At a higher speed than I had ever ridden before, the automobile raced through the streets of San Francisco, climbed up
and down steep hills, and dodged cable cars. Our destination,
an imposing three-story townhouse, rested atop a flight of
high steps. The first floor housed church meeting rooms, and
the family lived on the upper floors.

The family kindly prepared brown rice for me. I was also

treated to cantaloupe, which I had for the first time. It was so delicious. The melon's sweetness immediately relaxed me after weeks of hard rye crackers and roasted rice. I excused myself to take a nap and ended up sleeping the whole day.

My stay in San Francisco was a pleasant one. Over the next few days, my hosts took me to Golden Gate Park, Nob Hill, Fisherman's Wharf, and some Japanese gardens. When it was time to leave, they saw me off at the bus station, putting me right back of the driver's seat and explaining to him that I didn't speak English. On the journey, someone on the bus always looked after me, taking me to the rest room and making sure that I was comfortable.

From San Francisco, the bus traveled to Sacramento, the provincial capital. I marveled at the beautiful flowers along the way and the residents, attired in colorful summer clothing, sitting on the front porches by quiet tree-lined streets. Eventually the lush California countryside gave way to the hot deserts of Nevada and Utah. I had never seen such expanses of sand before. The Great Salt Lake dwarfed the big bay near the Izumo Shrine and Lake Biwa near Kyoto. I composed many poems in my notebook. The cathedral in Salt Lake City made a lasting impression on me.

> In the hot, noonday summer sun of the Rocky Mountains
> and Salt Lake,
> The lofty Mormon temple
> Reaches up toward heaven.

In Denver, another Seventh Day Adventist minister of Japanese descent met me. I enjoyed a vegetarian meal with him. At a coffee shop, he introduced me to Postum, a cereal grain coffee substitute that was then popular. During rest stops along the way, I once bought a package of bread. It tasted funny, and I realized it must have sugar in it. Before reboarding, I left the whole loaf on a bench.

In Nebraska, I heard someone in the bus singing Japanese songs. It turned out to be an American who had been in Japan right after the war. We talked a little. Fields of corn stretched endlessly in all directions as the bus rolled down the highway. I felt very much at home amid the ripening grain but had never seen such vast farms before. Once, the bus stopped to let deer cross the road at night. I wrote a poem about seeing the graceful creatures silhouetted in the headlights.

The next morning, I alighted at the next big city, which I thought was Chicago but turned out to be Omaha. By the time I discovered my mistake, the bus had left. Someone kindly guided me to an Oriental restaurant, where I met a Chinese lady who could speak some Japanese. She offered me some refreshments and put me on the next bus to Chicago.

Meeting Michio in New York

Mr. Shinohara, a student at the Maison Ignoramus who had come to America several months before me, met me at the bus station in Chicago. I accompanied him to the home of a Japanese family where he was staying and spent a couple days seeing Lake Michigan and some of the sights of America's second largest city. From there I took the bus to New York and was told to stay aboard until the last stop. Michio was waiting for me at Grand Central Station, the second to last stop. Eventually, he realized what must have happened and hurried over to the East Side Terminal.

We met at the Greyhound Bus Station and said hello. My first impression of him was that he was tall and skinny. I don't know what he thought of me, but I had been given a fancy lady's hat in Chicago which partially concealed my own short and skinny stature. Outside, a strong sun shone on Manhattan, and I felt that Michio would melt struggling with my luggage. I had two pieces of baggage, a traditional Japanese suitcase made from the netting of a willow tree and a big package of poetry books, writing materials, and sundries wrapped and tied in a scarf. I felt sorry my bags were so heavy and would have shouldered them myself since it appeared I was stronger than he was. But I noticed that in this country the men carried while the ladies waited, so I kept my thoughts under my hat.

After hailing a cab, we drove to the Columbia University
area. Michio was renting a room in an apartment on 103rd
St., between Amsterdam and Columbus Avenues. The room
had an upright piano, which he would occasionally play on it
though he had no formal training. I stayed in another room
in the same apartment. Michio's rent was $6 a month, mine
a little bit less. For the first time in my life, I was given
a house key—actually two keys, one for the downstairs entry
way and one for the apartment upstairs. Strange feelings of
isolation and fear came over me. It was so very different from
my home in Yokota, my college dormitory, and the Maison
Ignoramus where we had no keys or locks and everyone was
friendly and greeted each other.

After enrolling in Columbia graduate school, Michio spent
most of his time in the dark lower basement of the library
researching utopian proposals through the ages, from Plato
to the League of Nations. He typed them out in a study carrel
with two fingers on a second-hand typewriter. In the beginning
he had attended classes but couldn't understand spoken English
very well and tried to copy the notes of the person next to
him. But the other student was also a foreigner and having
trouble too. Realizing that it was fruitless to take classes until
his English improved, Michio started studying on his own.
From time to time, he worked at part-time jobs. When I
arrived, he was being supported by a Japanese restaurant
owner who shared his enthusiasm for world order.

One of the first places Michio took me to was a coffee shop
on Broadway. There I tasted coffee for the first time and as
we talked noticed a swelling in my legs. I couldn't walk, and
we had to take a taxi home. In the cab I took off my shoes
for relief. A week later I had coffee again and experienced
the same symptoms. I have never had it since. Another time
I took a sip of Coca-Cola. It tasted like funny herbal medicine.
In Japan I had eaten ice cream twice. The first time was at a
teachers' seminar in Izumo where I had a scoop of vanilla.
But since becoming macrobiotic, I didn't touch ice cream and
continued to avoid it in America. I also stayed away from

milk but tried cheese. Hokkaido had begun to produce cheese, and in comic books I had seen pictures of Swiss cheese with cute little mice frolicking in the holes. I especially liked grilled cheese sandwiches and continued to eat them occasionally until George Ohsawa told me to quit on his first visit to New York in 1959. Hot dogs and hamburgers had no attraction for me, and to this day I haven't tasted them.

After getting settled and sampling some forbidden foods, the first order of business was to find a job and learn English. Before leaving Japan, George Ohsawa told me the main thing to do in America was master the language. After three years, he proposed that we meet together at a world government congress in Paris. He gave me an English textbook, and I had begun to study it on the boat and bus. In college, we had studied English before the war. But we had no native English-speaking teachers, and except for a few words such as "yes," "no," and "thank you," I couldn't speak or understand it at all.

One day along Broadway Avenue, I went to a dime store, carrying the English book that George Ohsawa had given me by my side. We didn't have such novelty stores in Japan, and I was fascinated. With images of so many interesting things running through my mind, it wasn't until several blocks later that I realized I had left my English book behind. I ran back to the five-and-ten but couldn't find it. I was so ashamed. I had lost my teacher's gift. Ever after, I felt awkward in my study of the language and felt losing the book symbolized my failure to master American speech.

A Japanese employment agency on 42nd Street found me a live-in housekeeping job on the East Side. I moved my few things to a spacious six-story townhouse on Fifth Avenue at about 96th St. My duties included cleaning and cooking. I was supposed to cook dinner for my employers, Mr. and Mrs. Singstead and their son, but I didn't know how to prepare meat. Mrs. Singstead got angry and said she would do it herself. While cleaning the kitchen, I found something in the pantry that looked like sesame butter. It was peanut butter.

I lived on that, bread, and oatmeal. My eating habits were so simple and cheap, I think that is why they kept me as long as they did.

To make up for the loss of my English text, I bought the children's book, *Bambi*, in a drugstore. It had colorful illustrations and big, easy-to-read type. One day my employer came to my room and found me reading about Bambi.

"There are no Bambi here," she said indignantly, looking under the bed and in the closet to indicate that there were no deer in Manhattan.

"You must study this instead." She handed me a big cookbook with recipes for stews, roasts, and fondues.

Another time, in mid-August, a military parade came up Fifth Avenue. I rushed to the window to watch the marching band and long files of smartly-dressed soldiers. Mrs. Singstead came in the room and scolded me, "Don't watch the parade. Your job is to clean."

But I couldn't concentrate on my work and a few minutes later was back at the window. She caught me again and under her stern gaze I went back to my duties.

The parade reminded me of the autumn festival in Yokota, when horses and cows from the surrounding valley would be driven to market. When the animals passed the elementary school where I was teaching, I would reprimand the children who wanted to watch, "Don't go to the window. You must study." Now someone was admonishing me in the same way. I felt sorry for the children and realized that I was now reaping what I had sown.

Normally, I started work about 8 A.M. But it was confining being in the apartment all day. One morning, I woke up early and snuck out to Central Park, on the other side of Fifth Avenue. At 5 A.M., the peace and quiet of the park reminded me of the Izumo countryside. I took off my shoes and stockings and just like Julie Anderson in *Sound of Music* sang and danced on the grass. The early morning dew on my bare feet felt exhilarating after nearly a month of travel and city pavement. I returned to the townhouse barefoot. The doorman was

shocked at my appearance and ushered me inside quickly
before I was spotted. I went out to Central Park the next
several mornings. One time I walked up to 110th St. where
there was a lovely pond. I observed a strange gentleman
following me. When I walked, he walked. When I stopped,
he stopped. Fear overcame me, and I realized I wasn't in the
countryside any longer. That experience ended my strolls
before sunrise.

Chicago Sojourn

The first month I made $100, a small fortune in those days.
But my visa had expired. Michio felt it was better for me to
go to Chicago to get an extention. There was a larger Japanese community there than in New York, and friends in
Chicago could probably help me. On the way, we stopped in
Cincinnati to visit Florence La Fontaine Randall. She had been
corresponding with George Ohsawa and had helped translate
Jack and Yo-yo in Alice-Land into English. He would often
read her letters to us in Hiyoshi, noting wryly, "Study her
writing well and you will learn how to write love letters in
English." Once she had sent Lima and the girls at M.I. some
lovely European-style dresses. We all tried them on and had
our picture taken, with the tallest Darbin at one end and, as
I recall, Sidonie or Agnes, the shortest, at the other.

Florence lived on a farm with her husband. I was surprised
to see that the bathroom was located outside, just like in
a traditional Japanese farmhouse. I thanked her for the dresses
she sent and left her with a kimono.

In Chicago, a room was waiting for me with the family
I had originally visited. In September I enrolled in beginning
English conversation classes at a University of Illinois building on Navy Pier. I took a housekeeping job in a penthouse
on State Street. My employers, an Armenian couple, had
a carpet factory or warehouse. The husband was away most
of the time managing the business. The wife, a very tall,
beautiful lady, remained at home, taking piano and singing

lessons. She also had a driver, a cook, and another house-keeper. My job was to bring her breakfast each morning in her room and to keep the kitchen clean. During the day, I attended classes. The view from my window was very beautiful, taking in the waterfront and sky.

For George Ohsawa's sixtieth birthday, October 17, I sent a letter to the M.I.:

> Happy Birthday, my dear Papa,
> Under a chilly and cold Chicago sky, my memory of you is coming back. I recall the strong, vibrant colors of autumn in Hiyoshi and the wind blowing through the grass in the garden. Last year at this time, I remember you opened your presents with a smile, protesting, "I don't need any gifts. The greatest present you can give me is your strong commitment to spreading the macrobiotic way of life." I clearly recall these words of yours. I have nothing more to ask for now. I just look back, missing everyone and with tears coming to my eyes. May my wishes for you be just one drop of oil in the fire of your birthday candle.

*

> Dear Lima,
> I think your empty wallet is getting emptier. I can hear the bell of a church ringing in the distance. I'm celebrating Papa's birthday alone. I have fond memories of last year's party. I insisted that André contribute to the expenses of the celebration and also Augustine, even though he was in Paris. . . . Please have a wonderful birthday party for George. It's marvelous for everyone to be able to listen to his lectures in person. I already feel as if I left Japan a long time ago. Living alone, I feel I am now way behind everyone else in my studies. Yet as many students as possible there should go out into the world. That idea is always in my heart. I would like to do something for all our friends who go forth, such as

contributing to travel expenses and securing letters of guarantee. Someday I hope I will be able to help others in this way. Thank you, Lima, for everything you have done to make my journey possible.

I enclosed personal notes to some of the students at the dormitory. To Sidonie, I recounted my reception by some Japanese-American ladies in Chicago:

Today I went to teach Japanese at Mrs. Nishimura's house. It was my first class. I led everyone in singing "The Acorn Song," a children's song I used to teach my kindergarten class in Yokota. After class, one of the Japanese ladies invited me into the next room. They brought out an assortment of winter coats and clothing for me to try on. Since it was used apparel, they hesitated but expressed hope that I would like it. I was very happy. I tried each one on, and to my delight they were just my size. Also last week while walking together to work, Mrs. Shirokawa gave me a green mid-length coat, a black scarf, and a brown suit with a gray and dark green scarf. Today's assortment was similar and in the styles and colors I loved. There was a white blouse, very elegant, with a scarf. I said they did not know me very well and I was not qualified to accept such beautiful gifts. That evening, I walked home to my room with a heavy box of dresses, which I hugged close to keep me warm. There are really too many clothes for me to wear, and I'd like to send some of them to you in Japan, if I can.

In a note to Alcan Yamaguchi, the boy who had once slapped me for my unladylike behavior, I commented on the *Manyōshu*, the anthology of classic Japanese poetry:

It is said that the beauty of the *Manyōshu* comes from unknown authors who themselves didn't know how to write. This is a theory I agree with whole-heartedly.

Of course, it is very convenient to be able to write. But if we stick just to writing, we may lose some of the poetic sound and sense of words. In the old days, people copied down everything by hand. Nowadays, we have a big publications industry, and words have become dead.

From my letters you must think that I'm very strict in my macrobiotic practice. Perhaps my writings give that feeling. I eat whatever is available. I am watching my condition, controlling myself, and always thinking according to yin and yang.

To Bertrand, I described my first impressions of Michio:

From Michio, I am learning to feel a great yearning for humanity. He feels that the human race is sinking down in a deep pond without a bottom. He hopes to stop it with world government. He talks passionately about a new world order and really devotes all his energies to this cause. When I was in New York, he wrote an article about the future entitled "1960." In English, he subtitled it "Nostalgia of Humanity."

You asked me what he is doing. I can reply to you from what I have observed. He really is someone who has deep love and wishes to save the whole of humanity. He is always talking about the fate of the world and he likes to sit American-style in a chair. Once we went to the Catskill mountains to visit the countryside. He tried to avoid stepping on the roadside grasses and commented that we should not kill the smallest fly or mosquito. I have always loved to pick wild flowers, and he was sad when I took their lives in this way. Other times he criticizes human folly very bitterly. He is sentimental but also has this other side to him. He really wants to change the world and has confidence that it can be changed. I think he can do it. That's Michio.

To Libéral, I enclosed some of my first impressions of

New York City. In the big cities of America I realized I couldn't write poetry anymore. The well-spring of my inspiration had completely dried up:

> God created day and night, but with the invention of electricity and artificial light, human beings have violated and destroyed the real meaning of night. New York really has no night. The original deep, quiet, spiritual feeling of darkness has been lost. If we no longer experience the solitude and mystery of the night, how can we appreciate the brightness and radiance of the sun? Night is a time of resurrection. In darkness, we quietly take our rest. I can imagine people living such powerful lives in olden days when it was truly dark, and I miss it.
>
> Human life is said to have originated in the Pamir mountains of Kashmir. I dream of visiting the Himalayas someday, but don't know when I will be able to do so. Maybe I will travel to Europe and get a chance to pass through the Ural mountains in Russia. I would like to be somewhere in a very quiet, deep forest, contemplating Buddha and Jesus. Let's sing "Old Lang Syne" together again.

In early fall, I received a deportation notice from Immigration. I didn't understand what it meant and called Michio in New York. He said it was very important and arranged for Japanese friends in Chicago to help me, but they were not successful. One day I went to the Immigration office by the Michigan Avenue Bridge. An official told me my visa had expired and I could no longer stay in the country. I cried and told him I wanted to stay. He just laughed at my teary outburst and took away my passport. He also took my fingerprints. I was terribly shocked. I had read about criminals being fingerprinted. But I had never been arrested before and couldn't understand what awful things I had done. I wept all the way back.

I didn't know what to do and decided to remain in America until I was compelled to leave. Meanwhile, I resolved to earn as much money as I could in case I had to travel. I quit my English classes and started working at a restaurant owned by a Japanese family. It served American-style food, and I was hired to help serve breakfast, from midnight to 5 A.M. But the graveyard shift proved too much. Through a friend, I got another job in the warehouse of McGraw-Hill publishers, where several Japanese were working. My job was to bring baskets of books from the shelves to fill orders.

With a little money coming in, I could now afford a place of my own and rented a room in the Japanese Buddhist Academy. There were no cooking facilities there. I ate mostly instant Quaker Oats, which I heated with hot water from the tub and a little salt. For lunch I took Norwegian flatbread and Nabisco biscuits. Except for Postum, there was nothing I could order in the employee cafeteria. I supplemented my meals with whole wheat bread crusts from the restaurant I used to work at. I observed that the edges of sandwiches were neatly trimmed and thrown away. The old Japanese gentleman who owned the restaurant was happy to save them for me.

Work at McGraw-Hill was intense, from 8 in the morning till 5 at night. On Christmas Day, I worked an hour overtime and earned a little more money. I began to notice that my condition was tired and intestines sluggish. Instead of taking the bus to work, I decided to walk and everyday began walking or running the eleven or twelve blocks to work and back along the lakefront. The exercise made me stronger and also helped protect against the cold.

At the Buddhist Academy, a priest kept asking me why I was making life difficult for myself. "In Japan, you could have a nice job or get married and have a family," he said. "It is unnecessary for you to be here." None of my answers satisfied him. My attitude toward America was positive right from the start. In Japan, we have a word, *ikoku*, which refers to strange countries. Yet even crossing the desert, I felt an intimate feeling of kinship with the land. The natural beauty of

Central Park and Lake Michigan was not foreign to me. Once Michio and I visited a Jewish temple in Brooklyn. The songs were very beautiful. They reminded me of temple music in Japan, and I felt as if I was in an ancient Shintō shrine. "Why do we call America a foreign country?" I thought. "The world is really one."

Dream and Shadow

As the autumn leaves began to fall, I felt increasingly lonely apart from Michio. In New York, we had grown very close, complementing and intuitively understanding one another. I liked his nice, gentle manner, earnest dedication to his studies, and merry sense of humor. In turn, he seemed to appreciate my quiet disposition, initiative, and perseverance. But because of our poor material circumstances and uncertain immigration status, it was not realistic to think of settling down. I knew that his life was completely devoted to world government and world peace, and I felt content just following in his steps.

In America, I observed that relations between the sexes were much more casual than back home. Traditionally Japanese boys and girls were brought up separately, which helped to increase attraction on both sides. In this country, boys and girls were always together, studying, sitting, and talking —without any special feelings developing between them. For us, it was customary growing up for groups of girls to relate to groups of boys, but for a single girl to be alone with a single boy was very uncomfortable. For the first time, with Michio, I began to overcome these feelings.

In Chicago, the greater my difficulties and loneliness, the more my love for people grew. I began to understand the spirit of Basho, Lord Byron, and other itinerant poets whose work I admired.

> In the dusk of hoary winter,
> By the side of the frozen lake, I am alone.

The sun is so faint
I lack even a shadow for a companion.
I have no warm evening meal waiting.
I have no one to talk to.
I don't know how to express my sadness.
From deep inside, I feel love well up.
In the corridors of my memory,
I meet Mother, far away friends, and many people.
Now I would like to embrace you all.
From such sad wanderings,
Eternal love springs.

I enclosed some of my poems with a letter to the Ohsawas:

Dear George and Lima,

Thank you very much for worrying about me. I've become a little yin, but am still OK. Through the efforts of many friends, I have begun my travels. At the same time, I feel very sad and am experiencing the ephemerality of life. I've met many types of people and experienced many different situations. Things change very quickly. Everything looks complicated, but I can see that it is nothing but my dream and shadow. . . .

I see everyone's health, spirit, constitution, and way of thinking are all one. I watch very carefully and observe the secret of food. The compass of yin and yang is really fun to use. Of course, my understanding is very immature. But I can't think in any other way now.

A couple days ago I sent a small New Year's gift to everyone. I'm sorry if it doesn't reach you in time for the New Year's seminar. It is a comic book, *The World That Isn't*, by Frank Tashlin. A satirical look at society, its theme is similar to Michio's article "Dream and Shadow" in *Le Compas*. I hope you all enjoy it.

Many times, during my difficulties in Chicago or walking along the dark streets in New York, I would think back to

my happiest days teaching in Maki. Sometimes when I closed
my eyes, I could see clearly the golden color of the rice fields,
the beautiful autumn sky, and the proud mountain ranges of
Izumo. But most of all I could see the shining, happy faces of
my pupils as they splashed in the mountain streams, quietly
composed drawings in the classroom, or recited their haiku.
These memories became the source of my life energy and at
the same time created an endless dream. I wanted to share and
give away to everyone the small joys and happinesses we had
experienced together.

From New York, Michio sent me the copy of another article
he sent to Japan. After reading George Ohsawa's translation
of *Man the Unknown* by French scientist Alexis Carrel,
Michio's understanding of macrobiotics deepened:

> After reading *Man the Unknown*, I have found that the
> Unique Principle is really the absolute law of the uni-
> verse. That I now really understand deeply. I have told
> hundreds of people here how important correct food is.
> From this foundation, all of life's problems develop,
> indeed life itself. I can feel confidence developing from
> deep within. Our way of life is really grounded in truth.
> For human prosperity and survival, we must dedicate
> ourselves to spreading our message. Everything, in-
> cluding the structure of society, war and peace, sickness
> and health, wealth and poverty, are created by food and
> environment. World government is only part of that
> creation.
>
> What is reality? Everything in the universe is spiralling
> around a central vacuum. This spiral unfolds according to
> the Order of the Universe. It is the highest law of human
> beings. Reality is nothing but the Order of the Universe
> itself. I really understand now how my thinking and
> theories are completely encompassed by the Unique
> Principle. The target of world government is very short
> in comparison to the deep, long human balance achieved
> by harmonizing with the Order of the Universe.

My spirit is burning with this insight. How to explain it to people is the biggest goal of my life. I think I need more study and experience of life. I need your help in understanding the nature of food, environment, peace, and human development. Questions continually rise from my innermost heart. Now I feel confident that I can solve them. It is really surprising. Recalling my former studies and direction, I realized I just followed what I had been taught by modern education. But this year, the edifice of my past learning lies demolished and broken. Law and politics, social and moral education, history and economics—these high towers now stand empty for me. Graduate school and university research depends on modern science. It's like Jesus amid the Pharisees and Sadducees. Students are writing details from rote memory, acquiring degrees, and seeking status. But all those things are just appearances. To my eyes, they are all manifestations of ignorance and hopelessness. I can now see these things.

Since 1949 my daily food pattern has gradually begun to change. At the end of this year, I now have confidence that I can tell everyone without any hesitation about my daily way of eating. Animal food has almost disappeared from my diet. Sometimes I have a little milk, but it too is declining. I enjoy dark pumpernickel bread and hope it's good quality. It becomes hard in a few days, so I chew very well, making it soft with saliva.

Return to New York

At the end of the year, Mitsuko Yodono, the friend who introduced me to macrobiotics, came to visit me in Chicago on her way to Brazil. Meanwhile, my passport was returned, only to expire. To renew it, I had to go to New York. There was no Japanese Embassy or Consulate at that time because of the Occupation, just a Japanese Overseas Agency. I packed my bags, which had grown heavier with the acquisition of a typewriter, and with Mitsuko returned to New York. I was happy to see her again. She was as energetic and active as ever and took such large strides I had a hard time keeping up. We had Michio's room all to ourselves. He was in Tennessee, acting as guide to the mayor of Iwamizawa, Japan, who was visiting America enroute to a world peace congress.

From New York, I wrote George Ohsawa, bringing him up to date on my move. I described a dinner party in Chicago I attended with Mr. Shinohara, given by the United World Federalists. There were about sixty people present. Mr. Shinohara and I gave a short report about the Student World Government Association in Hiyoshi. George Ohsawa had published a poem in his most recent magazine which I especially liked:

> Until midnight the girls are selling
> The World Government newspaper on the streets.
> Without pause or rest, I write all night.

I told him how much I liked his article, "Disabled Soldiers and Peace," and how it really went to people's hearts, like Jesus cleansing the temple. Nobody dared to say what George Ohsawa said. He saw things clearly and warned without fear or favor. For the coming year, I told him that my four goals were 1) to try to stay in the United States for three years, 2) to invite Abe and other students at the M.I. to visit, 3) to help George Ohsawa obtain permission to leave Japan, and 4) to write and translate fairy tales.

In New York, the Japanese Overseas Agency had just moved from the Grand Central Station area to the Empire State Building. On the 72nd floor, I presented my passport to the officer behind the counter for a renewal. He admired my handwriting. He asked me to come to the office and help, and I took advantage of the opportunity to work immediately. My duties involved helping people extend their visas and passports. Many of these who came, like myself, had immigration problems. I secretly encouraged everyone despite their difficulties until the best solution revealed itself.

I moved back to the room adjacent to Michio's on 103rd St.

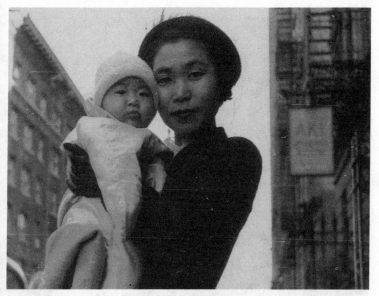

16.   Aveline and daughter Lilly in New York, 1953.

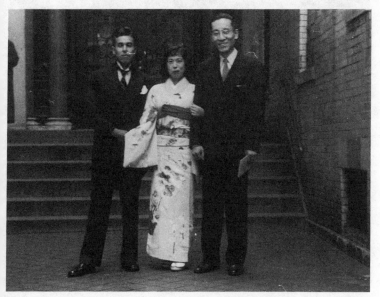

17.   Michio presides over wedding of Herman and Cornellia Aihara.

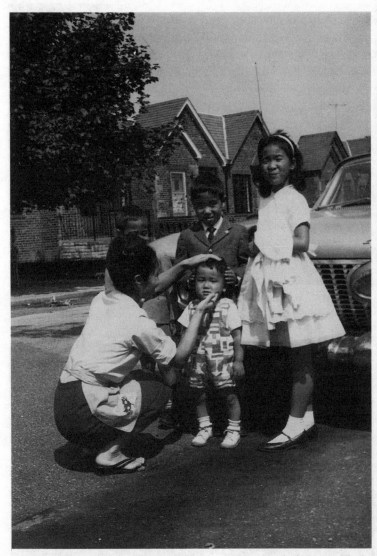

18. Aveline and her children in Queens, New York (Haruo, Norio, Lilly, and in front Phiya), 1962.

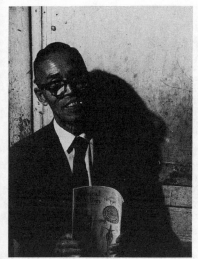

19.
George Ohsawa on a visit to
New York, early 1960s.

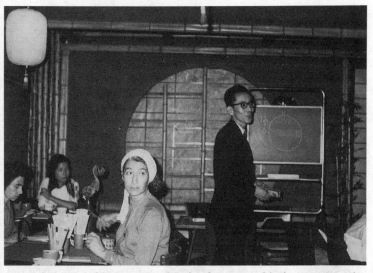

20. Michio teaching at Musubi, the first macrobiotic restaurant in
America.

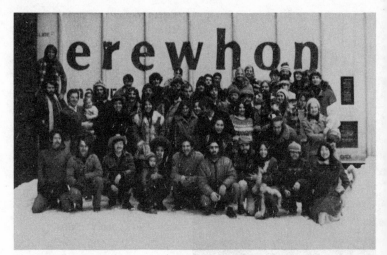

21. Erewhon employees during a snowstorm, early 1970s. (Aveline is in second row, beneath the "h".)

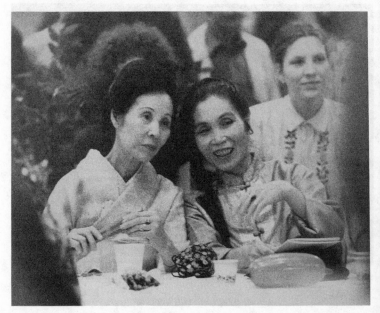

22. Lima Ohsawa and Aveline at a macrobiotic party in Boston, early 1970s.

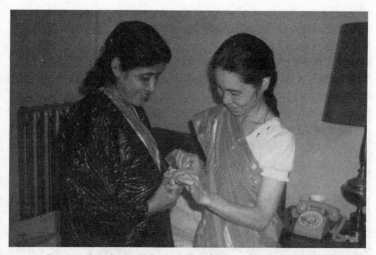

23. International Travels and Teachings: Learning to wear an Indian sari.

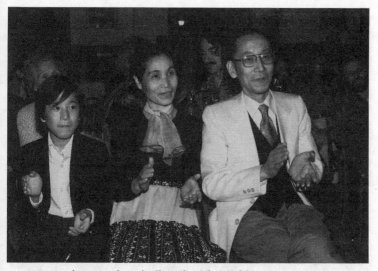

24. At a seminar in Brazil with Michio and son Hisao.

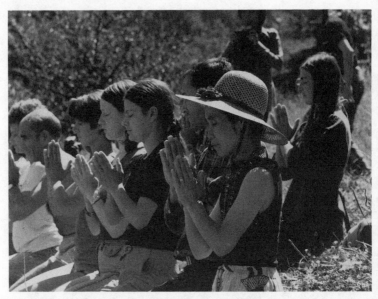

25. At a French palm healing class.

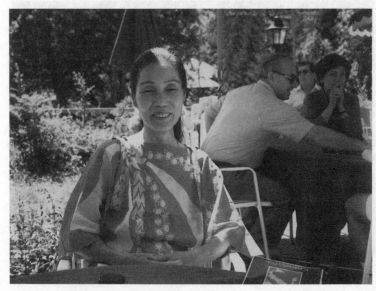

26. Relaxing in Switzerland after giving a cooking class.

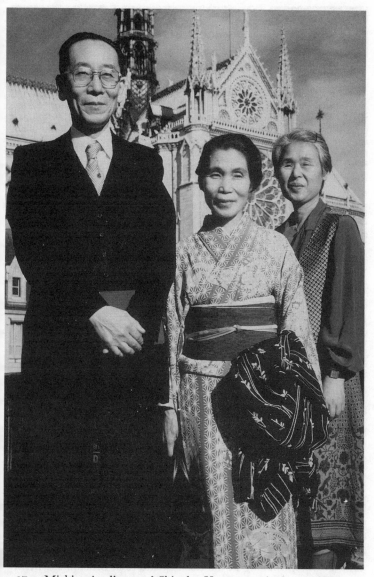

27. Michio, Aveline, and Shizuko Yamamoto in front of Notre
     Dame Cathedral in Paris.

160

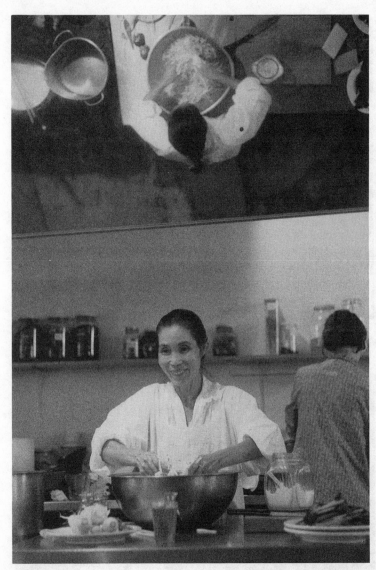

28. Teaching cooking at the Kushi Institute in Brookline. Mirror at top gives students overhead view of food being prepared.

Everyday I took the 8th Avenue subway to work. I remembered the rush hours on the trains in Tokyo, but they were nothing compared to those in New York. Everyone was so tall and the subway cars were so tightly packed that sometimes I couldn't touch the floor with my feet. Above ground, I came to appreciate the stunted trees and poor clumps of grass that grew amid the concrete.

Thursday nights I did housecleaning for a Japanese businessman. One night, I took a job behind the counter at a restaurant on 125th Street. It was a real greasy spoon, serving tongue of beef, livers and kidneys, and other strange meats. I couldn't stand it and quit after two or three nights.

Later that spring our landlord got married, and Michio and I had to find new rooms. On 119th Street, between Amsterdam Avenue and Morningside Drive, I found a large two-bedroom apartment. Located next to a Columbia dormitory and a small Japanese restaurant, it rented for $60. Michio found a room in the next building. My plan was to rent out the two bedrooms and do the cooking for my lodgers—just like a study house except I wouldn't be lecturing.

Japanese companies like Mitsubishi had just started to set up offices in New York for the first time since the end of the war. I called several places and advertised my services, including delicious Japanese food, especially noodles. One employee responded and moved in. I let out the other room to a Japanese at the university. On 106th Street, there was a small Japanese grocery store, and I would go there and stock up on soba, udon, nori, and whatever other traditional Far Eastern foods I could find. Through a friend in Chicago, I met Mr. and Mrs. Nakamura, who were interested in starting macrobiotics. Mrs. Nakamura came to my apartment sometimes and showed me how to prepare buckwheat groats. Kasha has a wonderful, nutty taste, and I loved it from the start. I also discovered wild rice and, though very expensive, loved to add small quantities to the commercially produced long-grain brown rice I was using. Through a small Japanese distributor, I found Hatcho miso, a traditional miso made from just soybeans and salt. I ordered a keg of this deep, savory miso from Japan, and it kept us in miso soup for almost a year. At this time, there was no good quality *shoyu* or tamari soy sauce so I just used salt and miso for seasoning.

My adventures with macrobiotic cooking began in this apartment. Our former place did not have cooking facilities, and we occasionally used the landlord's kitchen, but it wasn't very comfortable. Michio's way of eating at this time was rather haphazard as his letter quoted earlier suggests. He had not lived or eaten regularly at the dormitory in Hiyoshi, nor had George Ohsawa lectured much about the specifics of diet and food even when I was there. Also since he didn't cook much for himself, except for an occasional bowl of noodles or instant oatmeal, Michio tended to eat out, where good quality food was unavailable. Still, I observed that he did pretty well, enjoying grain products such as pasta and bread, vegetables, salads, and fish and seafood. But he also sometimes ate ice cream and foods with sugar. On these occasions, I would just sit quietly across the table at the restaurant and watch, not ordering anything myself. I couldn't see how anyone could eat sugar. To me, the beautiful cakes in America looked just like plastic. But I didn't say anything, confident that as his condition gradually improved his understanding of food would deepen.

I still continued to work at the Japanese Overseas Agency, which by now had been upgraded to a Consulate. One day, in late spring, I received a call and was told that my immigration case had been transferred from Chicago to New York. A hearing was scheduled, and I took a ferryboat to the immigration office on Staten Island. Passing the big Madonna in the harbor—the Statue of Liberty—I had feelings of impending imprisonment rather than freedom.

At the Immigration court, after a long wait, I was called in before a judge, several officers, and a stenographer. They asked me simple questions such as my name, nationality, and present address, but beyond that I couldn't understand their inquiries. They gave me a one-month extension and told me to come back with a translator.

A friend introduced me to a girl from Nagasaki who was studying at Columbia Teachers' College. She was unusually tall and big for a Japanese and had matriculated at a Catholic University in her hometown. A friend of her sister agreed to translate for me. At my second hearing, the judge asked, "Why don't you hire a lawyer to handle your case?"

"I have no money to pay a lawyer," I replied with the aid of this girl. "Instead I would rather leave voluntarily."

"Where would you like to go?"

"Paris," I said.

Then it occurred to me I might be able to come back. "When can I come back to the United States?" I asked.

"The next day," the judge laughed.

"Thank you very much," I smiled. I returned to my apartment with one more month's grace to make my departure.

Meanwhile, Michio's student visa had expired. He had to leave the country a short time earlier than I did. He decided to go to Europe too, first visiting London. We didn't know what the future would bring but agreed to try to meet. Since I had a lease on my apartment and hoped to come back, I sublet it to a young graduate of Keio University. He had come to America under the sponsorship of Frank Lloyd Wright, the famous architect, and spoke English well. Michio left on the *Queen Mary*, and I followed behind a week later on the *Queen Elizabeth*.

During my first year in America, I felt just like a dandelion floating across a field or an arrow in flight. Like Cinderella, I had been plucked out of the everyday world, scrubbing floors at the M.I. and dodging frowning station masters in Shinjuku, and set down in a new world of magic and wonder. I had no fears or anxieties about my odyssey and prepared to accept cheerfully whatever the future might bring.

8: Life in the West

"It is very difficult to know people and I don't think one can ever really know any but one's own country-men. For men and women are not only themselves; they are also the region in which they are born, the city apartment or the farm in which they learnt to walk, the games they played as children, the old wives' tales they have heard, the food they ate, the schools they attended, the sports they followed, the poets they read, and the God they believed in."
—W. Somerset Maugham, *The Razor's Edge*

THE *Queen Elizabeth* docked in Southampton, the port entry to London, after six days on the high seas. I gathered my things from a small cabin belowdecks and prepared to disembark. Two newsmen with cameras were waiting at the gangplank, and I looked around to see if there was some celebrity aboard. To my surprise, they crowded around me and took my picture. Somehow they had learned I was going to attend a World Government convention in London. In America, I had been struggling, working, lonely, and in trouble with Immigration. Suddenly, I was being treated as a visiting dignitary and photographed for a story in the next morning's *London Daily News*.

Officials of the World Government Association in London also greeted me and asked many questions. But I could not answer so well and told them I would like to introduce my friend, Michio Kushi, who was much more knowledgeable than I. I did not know where he was staying, but we had agreed to keep in touch through the Japanese Embassy. I went to the Embassy near Hyde Park. He had left his number with the staff. An official phoned him and said, "There's a Japanese girl here with a red dress and red shoes. Please come immediately." He came and took me back to his apartment near Bellside Park Square.

London still had a very dark feeling from the war. Trafalgar Square and other areas had not yet been restored and reminded me of bombed-out parts of Tokyo. I was impressed by the depth of the Underground and learned that much of the civilian population of the city had found safety there during the German air raids. In England, we visited Parliament, Buckingham Palace, Oxford University, and other sights. The fog was often so thick I couldn't see my hand when I held it straight out.

Michio conceived the idea of going to the Soviet Union to live and pursue his dream of world peace. Since Japan and Russia had not yet restored diplomatic relations, he could not get a visa. Undaunted, he decided to visit the Communist Party headquarters in London. Although his only interest was in studying society and human relations, they were impressed with his sincerity and said a secret visa might be arranged on the Continent.

My relationship with Michio deepened in London, and I appeared to be pregnant. But because neither of us had a permanent job or residence, it was still not practical to think about formally getting married. In our studies in Japan and travels abroad, we had come to see the foolishness of many laws and boundaries, customs and traditions, and didn't mind living together without legal sanction. Besides, I knew that our relationship was not primarily physical but based on a shared dream. In the old days, it was well known that arranged marriages lasted longer than fall-in-love marriages, because beauty and physical attraction faded whereas the spiritual qualities shared by the couple and their two families continued to grow and deepen. Although we had not been introduced in the customary way, we felt the dream we shared had brought us together. By encouraging my friendship with Michio through correspondence and by making arrangements

for me to come to America, George Ohsawa, our macrobiotic
family father, had served as matchmaker.

Around Christmas time, we left for Paris. The French
countryside was completely different than that of the United
States or England. The colors of the fields and mountains and
the texture of the soil reminded me of the François Millet
painting at my church in Yokota. In Paris we were welcomed
by Augustine, Gabon, and an Aikido teacher named Mochi-
zuki. The former Maison Ignoramus students had been the
first of Ohsawa's disciples to go abroad. In a nearby apartment, Madame Iwasaki, who founded a dressmaking school
in Yokohama, was living, and we visited her often.

During my pregnancy, I began to crave seaweed. One day,
I discovered some sea palm in the sidewalk fish markets. I
offered to buy it, but the vendors laughed and said it was just
for decoration. When I indicated I wanted to eat it, they gave
me the seaweed free. At the large outdoor food markets, we
also obtained many carrot and radish tops that were thrown
away and available for the taking.

Paris was much more beautiful than New York. During our
stay, we visited many cultural and religious sights. I especially
liked the Renaissance art at the Louvre. The spires of Notre
Dame Cathedral reminded me of the hunchback story by
Victor Hugo that I had read in college. Walking along the
Seine River and browsing among the bookstalls was always
very pleasant. Once we went to see the beautiful gardens and
exhibits of Versailles Palace.

In Paris, Michio again attempted to visit Russia, meeting
with various contacts he had been given in London. The final
plan called for him to go to Prague by train and there take
a clandestine flight to Moscow. But at the last moment
Michio changed his mind, and the train to Prague left without
him. He has said that if I hadn't followed him that morning
to the Paris station, the future of natural foods and holistic
health in America and Russia might have been entirely
reversed.

At the American Embassy I applied for and received a stu-

dent visa. Before leaving New York, I had been accepted at
Columbia University Teachers' College. Michio's visa was
also renewed, and in the early spring we made plans to return
to the United States. I came back first only to find that the
young man whom I sublet my apartment to wouldn't give it
back. While I was gone, Herman Aihara, a young engineering
student who studied with George Ohsawa, arrived and had
been ungraciously turned away by the temporary occupant.
I stayed at a friend's for several weeks until things were
straightened out and I got my apartment back.

Michio returned about a month later, and along with
Herman we set up our new household. With a new baby on
the way, Michio began to assume responsibility for me and
got a part-time job in Washington, D.C., as a guide and
interpreter at the State Department and Pentagon. He would
go to the nation's capital by train for several days to escort
visiting Japanese scientists and politicians. Once he went out
west to a nuclear energy and atomic-weapons site to serve as
an interpreter. Other times, he worked for big Japanese companies starting up business in New York.

Herman, who was very quiet and shy, worked at some
Japanese antique or gift store in Manhattan. Meanwhile, I
enrolled in conversational English classes at Columbia and
prepared meals for the two men plus different boarders we
took in.

Our apartment was located next to the Bachelor Hall of the
university. The apartment was very long, and all the windows
faced west except a few which faced north. We let out the two
bedrooms to Columbia students, Japanese businessmen, and
later to macrobiotic friends from the Maison Ignoramus in
Japan who moved to New York. The front dining and living
room Michio and I used for ourselves. Our furniture was
simple, mostly used: a bed, bookshelves, a writing desk, and
a square kitchen table. I cooked in the little kitchen, and we
often stayed up late discussing food, politics, and philosophy
with our boarders, guests, and friends. Looking back, I guess
it could be described as the first macrobiotic study house in
America.

During my pregnancy, I received another deportation notice.
I had a student visa but after one semester quit my studies at
Columbia to prepare for the baby. At the Immigration offices
on Staten Island, the officials questioned me again, but I still
had a hard time understanding English. They asked me when
I was born, and I said 1951. One officer made a funny face at
my reply. This time we hired a lawyer to represent me. He
was living in Brooklyn, and we became very good friends.
He argued before the hearing that that I shouldn't be deported
while I was pregnant. To everyone's surprise, we won the
case, and the immigration law was changed. Michio—a former
law student himself—was proud that we had changed the
American legal system, though it was a very tiny portion, for
the sake of human unity and advancement.

During my pregnancy, I had gone to Women's Hospital
at 110th St. and Central Park West for a check-up. A nurse
told me to take pills for an iron deficiency, but I didn't take
them. Back home in Japan, I used to watch Mother prepare
for the arrival of my younger brothers and sisters and missed
the assistance of a midwife. I could not resist the doctors when
it came time for the baby to be born. I could not tell them to
avoid giving me drugs because my English was so poor. They
gave me some sugar water, and I fell asleep for about a day.
When I woke up they brought in the baby. Then they gave
me an injection to kill the pain, but it produced a horrible
feeling, as if all my bones were being torn out. It was the
worst pain I have ever experienced. Later they gave me intra-
venous feedings of glucose in the arms. I fell asleep immediately after only one or two drops.

Our new daughter was named Lilly, after the Midori, the
beautiful wild lily I loved in the hills and mountains of Izumo,
my home province. I stayed in the hospital five or six days
and insisted on breastfeeding, though almost no American
women were doing so at the time. Michio was away on a trip
and came a couple of days later to the hospital. It was a wonderful experience for both of us.

At home, prior to the birth, I had started to buy patterns
at the dime store to make clothing. One day, along Amsterdam

Avenue, I came upon a Salvation Army thrift shop and was amazed at how nice and inexpensive everything was. I brought back a big package of baby clothing, washed everything in a big pot with boiling water, and ironed it. I was very happy. We had a hard time making ends meet, and I felt proud of my Salvation Army background.

In Japan, newborn babies always slept by the side of the mother. At home, I naturally put Lilly to my side in our double bed. One day the nurse from the hospital came and was shocked that we didn't have a separate bed for the baby. She emptied out the bottom drawer of a dresser for me to use. We put it on a small table near the bed and used it for awhile. Later we bought Lilly a little bed of her own. It had never occurred to us to have a separate sleeping place for her before the nurse's visit.

Our apartment was located on the third floor. The elevator made it convenient to go up and down. But there were five or six steep stone steps from the first floor to the street below. They were difficult to navigate with the baby carriage. A beautiful garden extended along one side of Columbia University. I loved to take the stroller there to watch the children playing.

To survive, we undertook many small business ventures. We set up a Japanese language bureau for translation and interpreting. It existed only in the Yellow Pages. The office was in our home. We got many translation jobs, and a friend brought wooden blockprints from Japan, which Herman particularly liked selling. These enterprises helped us get extensions on our visas. Across from the Empire State Building, we set up a small trading company office. It was called R. H. Brothers. The name was short for Reconstruction of Humanity by Brothers. It was located near R. H. Macy's, and many people thought we had some connection with the famous department store. R. H. Brothers' main business was exporting used nylon stockings. Michio and Herman would collect them from the trash and discarded cartons piled up in the garment district. They checked each pair of hose for holes. Those that were still good were sent to Japan.

One of our closest friends at this time was Yukiko Irwin. A Japanese-American student at Barnard College, she lived in a dormitory nearby. She came from an illustrious family. On her mother's side, her grandfather founded the East India Sugarcane Company, importing sugar to Japan, and visited the Imperial Palace many times during the Meiji era. Her grandfather was American. In Japan, Yukiko had studied macrobiotics briefly. She later married and gave shiatsu massage in New York.

Roman Sato, whose family had printed George Ohsawa's magazines and books, came to New York. He originally visited Los Angeles and intended to return home, but after visiting us in New York decided to stay. He didn't want to invest in R. H. Brothers but together with Michio and Herman opened Azuma, a small gift shop at 61st and Lexington Avenue. It carried many Oriental items, including ceramics and lacquerware. Roman handled the deliveries, Michio handled the paperwork and legal matters, and Herman managed the shop. During this period, Michio also opened Ginza, a gift shop at 9 W. 8th Street in Greenwich Village with some American friends and Kabuki, a gift shop at 44th St. near 5th Ave., with two Japanese artists, Mr. Takai and Miss Morino.

Michio's talent for business brought a promotion. Mr. Uehara, a representative of a famous Japanese textile company came to New York, and stayed with us. He really liked Michio and convinced Takashimaya, one of the oldest and biggest department stores in Japan, to open a branch in Manhattan. Michio, who was in his early thirties at the time, made all the financial and legal arrangements, negotiating leases with realtors, securing all necessary licences, and hiring a staff. As vice-president, Michio presided over the gala opening of the store on Fifth Avenue, on the corner of W. 46th St. He had overseen remodeling the building's inside and outside facade and received a prize from the Fifth Avenue merchants' association. On opening day, people were lined up for blocks. Unfortunately, the store was stocked with too many expensive items. It was like visiting a museum—very beautiful to look at—but not many people could afford to buy anything. Around that time, many Americans bought expensive Japanese things but not in New York.

Michio was good at initiating enterprises but did not really have a flair for administering them. Takashimaya soon changed its inventory and became fairly successful, but most of our own small business ventures were lucky to break even. In his free time Michio was always reading and writing about peace and world affairs. He wrote articles, essays, and drafts of books, most of which were not really finished or polished. Some were sent to Japan, and occasionally one would be published in some small world government publication. From the beginning of our life together, Michio would stay up late, often into the wee hours of the morning, reading and writing, and then get up late the next morning. I think this pattern began with him in graduate school.

About a year after Lilly was born, I got pregnant again, we decided to legally marry. One day we went to City Hall. I recall that it was springtime since I wore a very light coat, made of light material, but Michio thinks it was winter. The exact date we don't remember.

In the registration office, the city official asked us to raise our hands and promise to love, cherish, and obey each other. After we did this, he asked us to exchange rings. In Japan we don't use rings, and I knew nothing about this American custom. To my surprise, Michio took out two gold rings from his pocket. The official took them and put one on my finger. It was too small and went down just to the first knuckle. He put the other on Michio's finger. It was too loose. The official made a funny face, as if he had seen just about everything before except this. Anyway, the ceremony was finished and we were married. Later, I asked Michio where he got the rings because I wanted to exchange mine. He pointed out

a small store across the street nearby our apartment. I exchanged it for one that fit my finger exactly.

Raising a Family

While living in New York, I received news that my mother
was very sick with diabetes. I wanted to return home to be
with her, but we didn't have any money. It was hard enough
for us to pay the rent of $60 each month. Instead, I made an
overseas telephone call. I learned she was in the hospital and
had already passed away.

I had missed Mother a lot since coming to America. Before
she died, she seemed a long way away. But after her death,
I felt her spirit closer to me. I looked at Yokota, my home
village, differently after that, too. Still, I would often cry
in the kitchen thinking about Mother. Our children had
never met their grandmother and were too little to understand my sorrow.

During the four years I had been abroad, I had corresponded
with her occasionally. I didn't tell her about my husband until
after I was married. She was surprised. She didn't know what
kind of person I had chosen to spend my life with. She asked
why I hadn't contacted her before. Also, she once criticized me
in a letter for not resting after the birth of my children. In
Japan, the custom is to rest for at least one month after delivery, and for the first two weeks, the family takes complete
care of the children while the mother stays in bed resting
and recovering her strength. In my case, I did not have any
help, so I returned from the hospital after five days and began
to cook and work as usual. I wrote her a letter describing my
experience and telling her I felt fine. She wrote back, scolding
me, saying that I must take better care of myself, or maybe
not now, but in later years, I would notice that my strength
and vitality were diminishing.

I was very grateful for all that Mother had done for me and
my brothers and sisters growing up. Her whole life was spent
working very hard, helping her husband and bringing up her

children. Her constitution was not so strong as my father's but she had twelve pregnancies altogether. The doctor terminated the last one because she was too weak to carry. She outlived three of her children; eight survived. I appreciated her simple, practical nature and the natural environment in which she brought us up. A poem I wrote tried to capture her spirit.

In the early summer
When the long rains end
And sunshine returns,
My mother told me
Happiness is giving away
More than you receive.

Although she was not able to meet Michio or my children, George Ohsawa once visited her home in Yokota. She was so busy, and he said the house was a mess. But he could sense her love for her children. He was also impressed with my father's spirit. He said I succeeded him.

After coming to America, my husband kept in better touch with his parents than I did. When he told them we had married, they must have checked my background. I didn't know whether they were happy or not at his selection, but they wrote that my handwriting was very beautiful.

Raising a growing family in New York kept me busy. After Lilly came Norio, our first son, in 1953, then three more sons—Haruo in 1956, Yoshio in 1959, and Hisao in 1966. On weekends, we would make plans to take the children out to Riverside Park or some local spot, but Michio was invariably preoccupied with some peace or world government project. I would be ready after lunch, and the hours would tick away: 2 o'clock, 3 o'clock, 4 o'clock. Pretty soon it was too dark to go at all.

In 1959, a macrobiotic friend opened the Zen Teahouse in Greenwich Village. It served very simple food, tea, and snacks Alcan Yamaguchi, a student of George Ohsawa's, helped and did most of the cooking. This was followed by Musubi Restau-

rant, which opened in midtown near Carnegie Hall, on 56th
Street. Musubi served more substantial cooking, including
brown rice, miso soup, and various vegetables and seaweed.
Mr. Sato took the initiative for Musubi. Junsei Yamazaki, one
of Ohsawa's students, arrived from Japan and set up the first
rice cake machine at Musubi. It was operated by hand, producing four puffed cakes with each turn. We jumped up each
time they came out.

In 1959 George Ohsawa came to visit America for the
first time. Yoshio, my fourth child, had been born about
a month earlier, and I drove to the pier on the Hudson River
to meet his ocean liner. Some Japanese friends of ours had an
old greenish-blue Mercury, which they had to sell before
returning home. It was a big car and too good of a bargain
to pass up. Though neither Michio nor I knew how to drive,
we bought the car. With so many children to care for, it
would be a real convenience. We had moved from Manhattan
to Queens and were now living in the Regal Park area in
a rented one-family house near Woodhaven Boulevard. Things
were more spacious and spread out than near the Columbia
University campus.

I enrolled in an auto driving school but couldn't seem to
get the hang of it. At the time of the driver's test, the instructor said, "Do you really want to pass?"

I replied, "Yes."

"Then give me $75, but don't tell anyone, including your
husband."

I gave him the money. The written test consisted of five
questions. Although I had trouble comprehending written
English, the officer looked at me with a funny smile. Later,
when I was tested for parking, I parked way far from the
curb. The officer laughed, but I passed. For three years, I
didn't tell Michio how I obtained my driver's license.

Meanwhile, my husband figured that if I got a license, he
could master driving very easily. He got a learner's permit.
The first time out, I sat next to him to help, but I was nervous and couldn't sit still. I could see disaster coming and

yelled "Oh" in a big voice. Too late. He ended up in someone's bushes and couldn't back up. Fortunately the owner was
very kind and helped us push the big Mercury out of his
damaged shrubbery. Since then, Michio hasn't driven again.

Driving to the pier to meet George and Lima Ohsawa
brought back memories of living at the dormitory in Hiyoshi
and selling newspapers on the platforms in Tokyo. I had not
seen them in eight years. Shortly after returning to New York
from Paris in 1953, George had sent us a letter, notifying us
that his travel restrictions had finally been lifted and he would
like to come to America to visit. Michio, Herman, and the
other macrobiotic boys were scared at this prospect, since
they hadn't developed anything yet. They felt maybe it was
better that he postpone his visit. Many times the subject of
Papa's coming came up around the kitchen table and provoked
heated debate. Only I strongly wished George Ohsawa to
come, but he decided to go to India instead.

After a year in India, the Ohsawas journeyed to Africa,
where they visited Dr. Schweitzer's jungle hospital in Lam-
barene. There George Ohsawa contracted tropical ulcers and
became deathly ill. He had deliberately made himself sick in
order to prove to the great philosopher and medical doctor
that macrobiotics could relieve any illness. However, there was
little food there with which he was familiar that could be used
to reverse this agonizing condition. Michio and I read a letter
he sent us and felt he and Lima should leave Africa immediately. But we had no money to send him a ticket. One day,
on the New York subway, I saw a sign: "Fly Now, Pay
Later." I asked Michio what it meant.

"It means you pay little by little," he explained.

"That's wonderful," I exclaimed. "We can send him the
ticket now and pay later."

I asked Michio to call the travel agency, and they agreed
to write out a ticket for the Ohsawas in return for a down-
payment of $65 and the rest later. We immediately sent the
tickets, and Cornellia Aihara sent a package of brown rice and
strong, good quality Hatcho miso. The food helped George

Ohsawa to recover his strength, and the tickets enabled him
and Lima to get to Paris where they had many friends and
could fully recover. I was happy to help and overjoyed to
learn that they had flown to Paris and everything was well.
Now several years later, they were on their way to America
to see what their students had accomplished.

"Little Aveline, you are driving such a big car," George
Ohsawa said jauntily at the pier.

He was very pleased that I had come to pick him up myself,
along with Michio. The boat ride from France had been
pleasant, and both he and Lima looked well rested. We arranged for them to stay at the Buddhist Academy on Riverside Drive. George started to give lectures there and Lima
gave cooking classes. Many people came, and the Aiharas
and Mr. Sato helped us make arrangements.

After the Ohsawas' visit, people wanted regular macrobiotic
instruction. Michio started giving lectures in Manhattan once
a week, sometimes in a hotel or other rented space. I started
to teach cooking classes in my home in Queens. Because of my
difficulties with English, inexperience in cooking, and so many
babies to tend to, I was reluctant to try. Once I tried to make
buckwheat dumplings in soup. The dumplings all melted, and
I felt so ashamed. But my first students were kind and said
they enjoyed them anyway. Slowly my confidence grew, and
I offered my class once a week.

Meanwhile, our household continued to grow, with the
arrival of my younger brother, Kyū He came over from
Yokota and managed Ginza for us. He liked America so well
that he stayed and has been living in the metropolitan New
York area ever since. Mr. Tsuji, a friend of Michio's from
Akita, where his parents lived, and an accountant for Takashimaya department store, also stayed with us. The store was
now very successful, and Mr. Uehara, the representative of
Renown, a cosmetics firm, also lived with us for a while.

Our Queens home in Regal Park was a typical suburban
residence. Located on the corner of an intersection, the two-
story brick house had a lovely yard and hedges. Inside it had

a nice entranceway, big living room, dining room, three bed-rooms, and a kitchen. We collected the usual assortment of furnishings, such as sofas, tables, chairs, and paintings. I had a washing machine, which was handy, and I would hang the wash on the porch upstairs or outside to dry. Later on, we also had TV. Growing up, our children all spoke Japanese be-cause that is what my husband and I spoke among ourselves. But if they were to succeed at school it was clear they would have to speak good English. We bought the television to help them get started. Lilly, Norio, and Haruo did so wonderfully they quickly forgot Japanese, though they can still understand it. They loved to watch Micky Mouse and Donald Duck, Lassie, and Westerns on TV, and occasionally we would join them. At first we sent our children to the public schools but felt they were not so good. There was a private Lutheran school in our neighborhood, and later we sent them there.

The small but growing macrobiotic community in New York experienced its first major crisis in the spring of 1961. It was the time of the Berlin Crisis, and the threat of nuclear war cast a shadow over everyone's destiny. The Ohsawas had just returned briefly to New York from France. In his lectures George Ohsawa gave a very pessimistic report of East-West relations in Europe and encouraged people to move to a safer location in case of war.

After the Ohsawas left, things came to a head at a com-munity meeting held in a hotel, near Musubi Restaurant, on 56th Street. About sixty macrobiotic friends attended, vigor-ously discussing whether or not to leave New York. A small research committee reported that the Sacramento Valley north of San Francisco offered the best protection against radio-active fallout. A group of those present strongly urged that the whole macrobiotic community move to the West Coast. As chairman of the gathering, Michio was asked his view. He told the divided assembly that he had decided to remain in New York and leave only if the international situation continued to deteriorate.

Twelve families decided to leave for California. Led by

Herman and Cornellia Aihara, musician Bob Kennedy, and
Frenchman Lou Oules, they sold their extra belongings and
made plans to drive across the country. I agreed with Michio's
views about staying in New York but liked the idea of traveling across country. The caravan left in July, to much media
publicity, and several weeks later reached northern California.
Those who had made the exodus settled in Chico, a small city
in the Sacramento Valley. To their surprise, they discovered
the existence of another nuclear facility nearby, making the
area a prime target after all. However, to everyone's relief,
the Berlin Crisis subsided and tensions eased. Eventually the
Chico community formed Chico-San, a rice cake manufacturing
company, which turned into a major macrobiotic distributor.
They also started cooking classes, published materials by
George Ohsawa, and began an annual summer camp that
continues to this day. The next year, when he came back to
New York, George Ohsawa told us that we had done the
right thing to stay.

After the departure of the West Coast contingent, Michio
decided to concentrate more on education. Michio separated
from Azuma and Ginza. Roman Sato's brother came over
from Japan and helped with Azuma. Under their management
it prospered and now has five or six stores in the New York
area. Because everyone worked to support themselves, the
focus of our early macrobiotic education was on summer
camps, where we could gather and study together during vacation time. The first was held in South Hampton, Long
Island in 1960, followed by camps in the Catskills. The
Ohsawas, the Aiharas (until they went to California), and
other macrobiotic friends in New York taught at these gatherings with us, and we started to attract many ordinary Americans, especially young people.

Our first young American student was Robert Fulton, who
learned about macrobiotics at Musubi Restaurant. He was the
grandson of Robert Fulton, the inventor of the steamboat, and
a student at Harvard. He was also studying karate. A big,
tall, very serious boy, he attended our summer camp at Indian

Hill in the Hudson Valley, and we were impressed with his interest in Oriental philosophy. His eagerness helped me understand that I had something important to teach. For the first time, I realized I could teach about the Far East. Before that, I thought I could only teach children.

One day, Robert mentioned that if we really wanted to develop macrobiotics, we should find a more natural setting than New York City. He himself often visited his family on Martha's Vineyard, the large island off the coast of Cape Cod in Massachusetts. He invited me to see the island for myself and arranged a private plane to fly to Vineyard Haven. It was the first time in my life I had flown. I loved Martha's Vineyard, and Michio agreed that it would be an ideal place for the children. In March 1964, I took the four children and rented a house in Gay Head for $100 a month.

Life on Martha's Vineyard was idyllic. Lilly, Norio, and Haruo loved the public school, sang songs constantly, and let it be known that they didn't want to return to New York. The classroom was organized very much like a Japanese kindergarten and had only fifteen children. There was a small Indian community in Gay Head, and I became good friends with a Japanese woman who married an Indian. There was a small restaurant and inn there, and we met very nice people. I started giving cooking classes out of the small house we rented. Three or four students came at first, including a French teacher from Boston. Later, more people came for brief periods from New York and Boston. Robert Fulton and Ramsey Wood, another Harvard student, came to stay with us. Robert was very active, swimming every day, even in March when the water was very cold.

I cooked for everybody—brown rice every day, along with wild grasses and greens I picked up, including dandelions and chives. Robert, who was very strict, became very strong on these wild foods. His legs started to swell, and we encouraged him to eat apples or other things. But he refused, thinking it was not macrobiotic to eat desserts, fruits, or other yin foods. The pain in his leg increased. On a trip to Aspen, Colorado,

to visit his father, he took a glass of orange juice and the
swelling and pain immediately disappeared. Like a lot of
macrobiotic people in the beginning, he learned from his
conceptual mistakes.

While living on Martha's Vineyard, I was able to write
poetry again for the first time in many years. In Manhattan
and Queens, the source of my creativity dried up. But here,
in the quiet, beautiful setting I felt one again with nature.
I still have some of the poems I wrote that first spring.

> I don't know when I first dreamed
> To pick up wild spring grasses
> In the crisp New England air.
>
> *
>
> Darkness falls.
> The big ocean and the big sky melt together.
> I am standing on the New England shore.
>
> *
>
> When I stand very still,
> The sound of the crickets increases,
> And the peach tree blossoms so beautifully.
>
> *
>
> The Indian clay pottery
> Is made up of many warm colors,
> Yet radiates a melancholy sadness.
>
> *
>
> I gaze at the far white flowers
> At the end of the beach,
> As the lighthouse flickers on.

9: The Sprouting
of American Macrobiotics

"I think a war is the quickest and the most violent
cultural exchange. We were by curious chance taken
in the rapid current and thrown up on the shore of
the East Coast of the United States. New England
is a very severe, coarse, and rocky place. I do not
know when we will be able to take root here."
—Aveline Kushi to friends in Japan

ROBERT FULTON helped us over the next year or two as
we completed our move from New York to New
England. In Boston, he was teaching at the Matson
Academy of Karate and made arrangements for George
and Lima Ohsawa and Michio and myself to lecture there.
The martial arts center was located near Copley Square, on
Columbus Avenue. About forty to fifty people attended. The
head of the academy, George Matson, helped promote our
talk. It was the first macrobiotic gathering in Boston.

Our children loved Martha's Vineyard, but Michio and I
felt Boston was better suited for our long-term educational
activities. Martha's Vineyard was isolated and accessible only
by ferryboat or airplane. We decided to move to Boston.
Robert Fulton suggested we look for a place in Cambridge,
which was an educational center and magnet for young people
from around the country. We found a house in the northern
part of town at 101 Walden Street.

Michio went back to New York to wrap up his affairs.
While the children and I stayed on Martha's Vineyard, he
had begun teaching at the Genpei Restaurant, a small macro-

biotic eating place we set up in midtown Manhattan on W. 46th St. near 5th Ave. It was named after two medieval Japanese clans, the Genji and Heike, which fought a bloody civil war. We picked the name as a symbol of peace and reconciliation. The restaurant also tried to be a unifying force for New Yorkers. It served both white rice, which they were used to, and brown rice, which was unfamiliar to them but far healthier. Michio taught in the back. After selling the restaurant, we had as usual many debts to pay, not leaving very much left over for our move to Boston.

Changing Lifestyles

Several new friends came to stay with us in our new home in Cambridge. There was a middle-aged woman who ran a French academy in Copley Square. She had come to some of our activities on Martha's Vineyard. Then there was David Levin, a young computer programmer. There were no home computers then, and the whole field was very futuristic. One day he took me to a computer company in Belmont or Lexington and showed me five or six big computers in a single room. I was amazed. They looked like intestinal tubes. David was very active and had a quick mind. He made good money and supported us at that time. He later married a girl named Cecile, who served as the Ohsawas' secretary when they visited New York. Later they went to Japan where he worked as a computer engineer and she studied cooking with Lima at the Nippon C.I. They eventually separated, and Cecile set up a macrobiotic center in Los Angeles and is today a senior teacher and counselor.

Michio began lecturing out of our home and started to give consultations. He also gave shiatsu massage. I never knew he had studied shiatsu, but the people who came to see him enjoyed it very much. Slowly macrobiotics spread. One by one, people knocked on our door.

Mrs. Prentagas, one of our earliest supporters, was a member of the Ruhani Satsang, a society which followed the teachings of a yoga master from India. She brought about five to seven other disciples, both gentlemen and ladies, to attend our seminars and cooking classes.

In the early 1960s, Cambridge was a center for psychedelic drug experimentation. We didn't know anything about drugs when we arrived. Gradually we noticed that some of our students were involved in their use. A few were friendly with Richard Alpert, a psychology professor at Harvard who was introducing LSD and later became well known as Ram Dass. The way we learned about drugs was interesting. Our house had a small entranceway and a front window that allowed light in from the outside. When someone came in, the way the light fell on them I could see their aura. I began to notice that some young people's auras were very shallow and fuzzy. This was puzzling to me because after eating good macrobiotic food, most people's auras become strong and clear. In Japan, we had a proverb: "When someone is going to die, their aura becomes shallow." I was reminded of that saying.

About the same time, we noticed some of our young American friends saying to each other, "You don't need to take drugs. Brown rice makes you high." Michio and I were perplexed. We knew that if you ate balanced whole foods, your body grew solid and strong and your mind clear and calm, but we couldn't understand the meaning of "high." Some of our students had very big pupils in their eyes. In Japan we also say, "The pupils open as death nears." A very nice girl came and studied cooking with me. A couple months after she left, I heard that she had died. Her pupils were very dilated. We were sorry so many young friends during this time were attracted to harmful substances.

Another time someone living with us invited a friend from New York over. He was pretty weak, and we gave him good food and some exercises to do. A few days later, he died in our house. We were afraid. Later we found out the father, who was a diplomat, and relatives were not upset. On the contrary, they were very thankful that we had taken care of him during his last moments. He apparently had a drug

186

problem, and they had lost contact with the boy a long time ago. We were happy that they understood and appreciated our efforts.

My husband and I wanted serious students like those at MIT and Harvard. We were disappointed they didn't come. Most people who studied with us came originally from the West Coast. To our surprise, we attracted hippy, underground types. They were very disorderly and flouted tradition. But they were seeking something larger than themselves and deeper than could be experienced in the universities or conventional life. George Ohsawa, who was very disciplined and orderly, had a hard time understanding this generation. He saw their attitudes and behavior as "a deep sickness." We did too at first. But later we came to see that the counterculture was reacting against the extreme materialism of modern society. The hippies included some of the most adventurous and creative young people. We felt it was our responsibility to guide them and help them recover their health and dream in life. As years passed, many drug takers and peddlers stopped drugs and went on to become founders of the natural foods movement and macrobiotic leaders, bringing health and happiness to thousands of people.

In Cambridge, we were also introduced to the sexual revolution. One of the few Harvard graduates who came to visit us was named Alan. He had passed with the highest honors, winning a silver watch. A very beautiful boy, he proved to be an excellent dishwasher and helped us in the kitchen. I made him a kimono at Christmas, and one of the girls in our house fell in love with him. He was so popular that we couldn't believe it later when we heard he tried to commit suicide. I went to the hospital to visit him. Even though his girlfriend was standing nearby, he was crying, calling for his boyfriend. I was very shocked. I could not understand.

Zen Macrobiotics

To spread macrobiotics, we needed to make good food

available. When we had first arrived in America, there was
virtually no organic whole foods. The small health food
movement sold chiefly vitamins and supplements. In New
York, we shopped at Japanese, Chinese, and other ethnic
grocery stores as much as possible. The selection was limited,
the quality uncertain, and prices for specialty items high. One
of our macrobiotic friends began importing miso, tamari soy
sauce, and seaweed from Japan. In our dining room in Cambridge, we kept a small shelf of foods for our students. We
distributed everything at cost. In the basement, we set up
a packaging room. In the evenings or on weekends, my husband and I would spend hours pouring tamari from large
bottles into small ones, sometimes with the help of our children. We also made up small packages of miso, brown rice,
and other basics.

I started looking for a wider selection of grains and vegetables to cook with at home. I put the kids in the car and
drove around different parts of Boston. In a small store in
Brookline, I found some high quality grains from Balanced
Foods in New York. At a Japanese food store, I found some
Hatcho miso and azuki beans. At organic farms in Concord,
Massachusetts and in Vermont, I found some unchemicalized
produce. Walnut Acres, a Christian organic farm in Pennsylvania, offered some whole foods by mail order.

In our house, we used food from these far-flung sources for
daily cooking. My meals became more American in style. I
started cooking azuki beans Boston baked bean style in
a ceramic pot overnight. One morning, I went down to the
kitchen and discovered that the beans were all gone. I couldn't
figure out why. Had I put them away? The pot was empty.
Then Peter Magnuson, a tall, lanky boy staying with us,
came down the back stairway attired in a red nightgown. He
confessed sheepishly, "I couldn't stop eating your beans. They
were so delicious. I ate them all up. I'm sorry." I forgave
Peter but still missed those lost beans.

Dozens of people came to visit us in Cambridge. Some
moved into our house, offering to contribute to the rent or

help out with the household. Others came only to classes. We never asked anyone about their background. There was no entrance test or prerequisite for studying macrobiotics. We never tried to stop anyone from leaving. This was the traditional Confucian style of teaching, although it was really simplicity itself. There is a Far Eastern proverb, "Never refuse to accept anyone who comes and never try to stop anyone who leaves." The pattern of natural living we established in Cambridge was refined over the years but has continued until this day.

The Ohsawas' Visits

The Ohsawas came once a year to see us in America. George and Lima were now living in France. In New York, they had always come for the macrobiotic summer camp. One year they stayed with us for several months in Queens. George brought with him a European scientist who had escaped from the Nazis during the war. He was interested in transmutation of the atom. While Lima and I attended to the cooking, the men —George, Michio, and the professor—spent hours reviewing the periodic table of elements and conducting experiments.

The Ohsawas were happy with the gradual development of our teaching in New York and Boston. George was a businessman in the beginning too. He worked for a big import-export company for many years until he was able to support himself as an educator. In the United States, Ohsawa discussed natural foods development with us. Everywhere he went, he carried samples of good quality foods, and many people asked him to comment on their products. In California, he talked with a Japanese family of rice farmers, the Kōdas, and convinced them to make brown rice. It was not organic but still a big improvement over before.

The first time George Ohsawa came to visit us in Boston, we stayed with Robert Fulton's grandmother. She was living in an apartment on Commonwealth Avenue near the Public Garden. We showed George some maple syrup and asked his opinion. We were very interested in his judgment of the quality of this traditional New England sweetener. He had never tasted it before. Opening the jar, he swallowed a spoonful.

"Ah, sweet!" he exclaimed.

Everyone waited breathlessly. Was it yin or yang? Was it suitable for macrobiotic use?

George Ohsawa didn't say another word. Just "Ah!" He ate the whole bottle without comment. We watched in amazement.

At the end, he beamed, pronouncing it "very sweet."

Michio tells many funny stories about binging with George in the cafes and coffee shops of Harvard Square. Lima and I would stay home at these times, supervising the household and minding the children. Sometimes we would go out too. Once we went to an organic farm in Belmont. On the way back, we stopped at a fruit stand by the side of the road to buy peaches. Lima really liked the juicy New England varieties. Like George, she sometimes craved yin after eating so yangly for awhile. But she was always modest, eating only a very small volume.

During his younger days, George Ohsawa recommended a wider variety of food, including fish and seafood. As he grew older, he became more strict in his way of eating and his diet grew simpler. In the early 1960s, he published his first book in English and decided to call it *Zen Macrobiotics*. The Zen wave was just cresting. There were Zen Buddhism, Zen Beatniks, Zen Archery, Zen Tennis. George saw that many people were teaching and studying Zen. He felt that real Zen was impossible without macrobiotics. Traditionally, Zen monks in China and Japan ate simply, usually just brown rice, miso soup, vegetables, beans and their products, sea vegetables, pickles, and tea. Also, George's first lectures in America had been held at the Buddhist Academy in Manhattan.

George had a tendency to use popular trends to spread macrobiotics. During the 1930s and 1940s, he had capitalized on current sentiment to reach people. During the war, he wrote a pamphlet, "Who Is Really Demolishing Japan?" He recommended that Japanese soldiers eat good food to win the war more quickly. Many people thought he was an ultra-nationalist, though later he was accused of antiwar activities and sentenced to jail by the military authorities. At the Maison Ignoramus, I noticed he mixed his lectures with political rhetoric to attract socialists, communists, liberals, conservatives, nationalists, and internationalists. He used anything to spread macrobiotics. No matter what your target in life was, he would say, you could approach it more quickly by eating well and using the unifying principle.

Michio and I disagreed with him about linking the name Zen with macrobiotics. We felt it was too limiting. It was true that Zen practitioners were originally macrobiotic. But so too were other Buddhists, as well as Christians, Jews, Muslims, and members of other faiths. When the novelty of Zen wore off, we felt that macrobiotics would suffer. However, there was no arguing with George. He went ahead and used the title *Zen Macrobiotics*. For the next ten years, macrobiotics was associated with Zen. Zen temples in Japan and America complained. Controversies erupted. Many people came to our home or classes expecting a religious atmosphere. Michio was treated as a Zen master or guru. The more he protested that he was an ordinary person, the more convinced some people became that he was an enlightened master. His patience and humility were taken as the embodiment of Zen simplicity. I was teaching the Tea Ceremony at this time. It also had historic connections with Zen. An aura of spiritual mastery was transferred to me too. In truth, I was just an ordinary housewife, focused on getting the children to school, doing the laundry, and preparing the next meal. Eventually, the Zen label to macrobiotics wore off. Michio and I were relieved.

Challenge and Response

In autumn, 1964 I became pregnant. On previous occasions, I had gone to the Women's Hospital in New York to have my babies. In Boston, I went to Children's Hospital off Boylston St. in the Longwood area to have my condition checked. The doctors said the iron in my blood was low. They recommended medication, but I didn't take it. Later, some friends arranged for me to go to a hospital in Jamaica Plain for the delivery. During my first four pregnancies, I had medical assistance. I wished a natural delivery, but I couldn't get it since the doctors didn't understand.

This time I explained my wishes to the staff and they agreed to help. The doctors were very patient. When my fever started, one asked me three times, "Would you like to have medication?" but I said no. Everything went smoothly, and I found it a wonderful experience. Afterward, I was very relaxed and happy with the results. It was completely different than before. We named our new son Hisao. In the future, I began recommending natural childbirth to my students. However, I cautioned that they must have been eating very well for awhile, and it is important to eat well after the baby comes. Good food is really the key to recovery.

At the end of the year, the first direct challenge to our teaching arose. The Cambridge police accused my husband of practicing medicine without a license. The situation was complex. It originated in this way. One day one of the Ruhani Satsang members brought his son to hear Michio. Michio was giving a lecture about acupuncture and displaying the small, delicate needles used by practitioners. The son was mentally weak. Later, he visited his girlfriend and had sex. The Ruhanis practiced celibacy. Afterward, the son felt guilty and cut his penis. He went to the hospital emergency room. Then his mother got very upset because of the high medical expenses. She held the Ruhani group responsible and demanded that they pay the bills. They thought the boy had gotten the idea of hurting himself from the lecture on acupuncture. The police were called in to investigate. They couldn't understand my husband's teachings and thought they were medieval. For showing people how to stick pins and needles in themselves, they thought he was a sorcerer.

In truth, Michio was not practicing acupuncture. He was

just demonstrating how people in the Far East traditionally used it to relieve pain and stimulate energy. But then nobody outside of Chinatown knew anything about acupuncture. Five or six years later, everyone knew of it after relations with China improved. We were really surprised to find ourselves in the middle of this case, as the parents and friends of the boy filed charges and countercharges and the police thought we were practicing voodoo. A friend introduced us to a lawyer named Ginsberg. He represented us before the town of Cambridge. Meanwhile, many friends wrote letters to the court in our behalf. Although the charges against him were absurd, Michio did not want to defend himself. In principle, he no longer believed in the legal system of justice. He felt that ideally people should resolve their disputes peacefully. Also practically, we were still having immigration problems and didn't want to draw attention to ourselves and possibly be forced to leave the country. The authorities finally agreed to drop the case if we left Cambridge. We were grateful to Mr. Ginsberg for his help. Soon after this incident, one of our lady friends introduced us to another wonderful lawyer, Morris Kirsner. That was the beginning of our association and friendship with him. Over the last twenty years, he has been our chief lawyer and confidant.

The Birth of Erewhon

After promising to leave Cambridge, we looked hurriedly for somewhere to move. It was my introduction to real estate, an interest that would grow over the years. I looked at houses in Boston, Everett, and Nahant. In Nahant, on Boston's North Shore, there was a beautiful beach-front estate owned by the founder of the Singer Sewing Machine Company. I liked it a lot. Meanwhile, Michio located a house in Wellesley which was formerly the dormitory of a small girls' college. Our choices narrowed down to these two. For the sake of our children, we selected Wellesley because the school system was better. If I had used Nine Star Ki, a traditional Far

Eastern system of astrology and directionology, more at the
time, I wouldn't have gone west. East was better. But I didn't
think that then.

In Wellesley, we decided to do things as legally as possible and have good relations with the town. We already had
established the East West Institute out of our home in
Cambridge. Mr. Tamura, one of my former classmates at
George Ohsawa's school in Japan, visited us. He was an 8th
rank Aikido master. On one side of the room, I made a dōjō.
We couldn't afford Aikido tatami mats, so we bought heavy
canvas used in sailboats and put it around the top of regular
gymnasium cushions. Then I invited jūdo and karate teachers
and students to come from around New England for a demonstration. My husband talked about Oriental philosophy and
macrobiotics, and I performed the Tea Ceremony.

People came from all over to see this new martial art. Once
they listened to Michio, many of them came back to study life
philosophy and macrobiotics with us. Soon we had young
people of all kinds visiting us, including many hippies, antiwar
protesters, and blacks. They would appear at all hours of the
day and night, visiting our house as well as the dōjō and
parking their colorful cars, campers, and motorcycles along
the neighbors' spacious lawns.

Until then, we had not noticed how prim and proper Wellesley was. It wasn't long before the town officials came to
check up on us. They told us we could stay as a family but
could not distribute food or hold classes in our home. It was
clear that we did not fit into the neighborhood and that our
way of presentation was not very smart. After only three
months, we decided to move again.

In France, George Ohsawa heard of our difficulties. He sent
us a thousand dollars. "We need money badly too," he wrote,
"but you have difficulties now and may need money too."
His gift was a great help. Aside from our educational activities, we had a hard time making ends meet. Our children had
only one or two sets of clothing each—some mixed cotton/
poly shirts as 100 percent cotton was unavailable. While they

were at school every day, I would wash their clothes, hang them up to dry, and iron.

From Wellesley, we moved to Brookline, a lovely residential town with wide streets, spacious parks, and good schools. Enclosed on three sides by Boston, it was an oasis of peace and quiet in the center of a big city. We rented a house at 216 Gardner Road near the high school. Downtown, in the Back Bay section of Boston, we started looking for a small storefront to hold classes and distribute food to our students. We found a small shop on Newbury Street, a fashionable section of brownstone apartments that had been converted into boutiques, art galleries, and cafes. An antique store was next door on the north side of the corner of Fairfax Street.

In the back we partitioned off a storage and packing area. In the front there were several shelves and a desk. We would buy brown rice, beans, and other staples in bulk, pack them in the back, and put them out for sale on shelves in the front. On Thursday nights, we had lectures. Michio prepared his talks at home, usually on some introductory aspect of macrobiotics. In our kitchen in Brookline, I cooked rice, made rice balls, and brought them to the lecture for the students. In the beginning, only a handful of people came. After my husband spoke, I talked about cooking brown rice and distributed the rice balls.

Evan Root, a young man from New York who had lived with us in Wellesley, became the shop's first manager. Sometimes he would spend the entire morning or whole day talking about macrobiotics to someone who walked in off the street.

It soon became clear that we needed a name for our store. I immediately thought of Erewhon. George Ohsawa admired Samuel Butler's utopian novel of that name. Sir Thomas More first coined the term *utopia* in 1500. In Greek, it means "nowhere." More chose it to signify the location of the ideal society. Butler later wrote a satire about a mythical paradise of natural health and beauty. He called it Erewhon, which is "Nowhere" spelled backwards.

Michio immediately agreed with the name. I was very

proud. We liked the name Erewhon because it was founded
upon a deep understanding of the Order of the Universe.
About 70 percent of the people we met had never heard of
Erewhon, and we explained to them its meaning. The other
30 percent recognized it immediately, and we were very happy.
We also liked the name Erewhon (or Nowhere) because the
utopia we hoped to inspire was not to be found in any geographical location. Some nineteenth century utopian colonies
and twentieth century ashrams and communes strove to become perfected models for society as a whole. After World
War II and the atomic bombing of Hiroshima and Nagasaki,
it became clear that the world was one. No single country,
culture, community, or church could serve as the center. From
now on, we were all brothers and sisters of one planetary
family.

Further Challenges

Meanwhile, another challenge to macrobiotics developed.
Beth Ann Simon, a young woman living in New Jersey, read
Zen Macrobiotics. After experimenting with an all brown rice
diet, she grew thinner and thinner. Refusing medication, she
ultimately died. The case became a *cause célèbre*. Government
officials, medical doctors, and the national media condemned
macrobiotics. The FDA—the Food and Drug Administration—
was called in to investigate. The principal macrobiotic center
in New York—the Ohsawa Foundation—was closed down by
the authorities. Across the country, health food stores were
warned that they faced criminal prosecution for selling books
on diet or nutrition recommending foods for specific illnesses.
Dr. Frederick Stare, chairman of the nutrition department at
Harvard, wrote an article for *Ladies' Home Journal* on the
dangers of macrobiotics entitled "The Diet That Is Killing
Our Children."

What was the truth behind this tragic case? In *Zen Macrobiotics*, George Ohsawa described ten levels of the macrobiotic
diet, ranging from number −3 to number 7. The lower

numbers included less percentages of whole grains and vegetables and greater percentages of animal food. The higher numbers included more whole grains and vegetables and less animal food. At the top, the number 7 diet recommended 100 percent brown rice. In the book and his lectures, Ohsawa stated that eating only brown rice for ten days would heal practically any sickness. He said it would also bring spiritual benefits. Macrobiotics gained the reputation of being the all brown rice diet.

In truth, brown rice and other cereal grains are a wonderful, nourishing food. They have been used in the Orient and many other parts of the world for thousands of years for keeping daily health and for relieving sickness. However, brown rice or other grain is very rarely eaten only by itself. If so, it is then taken for usually no longer than ten days. And it is taken under the guidance of an experienced physician or spiritual teacher. If taken longer than that or without proper guidance, it can lead to serious imbalance. The person can become very tight physically and very rigid mentally. Such unfortunately is what happened to many young people who began experimenting with macrobiotics in the 1960s. Many of them were spiritual seekers, window-shopping among different yogis, swamis, and masters. Naturally they aspired to be sages. But instead of starting at the bottom, they started at the top. Meanwhile, there were very few macrobiotic cooks, no macrobiotic cookbooks, and almost no centers or classes to attend except in New York, Boston, and northern California.

As a result, misconceptions flourished about what macrobiotics was. Many mistakes in food selection and cooking were made. Some were serious. In Beth Ann's case, she reportedly had been experimenting with drugs and had not taken any cooking classes. She apparently did not know how to prepare grains and vegetables properly and ate far too narrowly. George Ohsawa later said that young American friends were foolish to start with the number 7 diet or stay on it beyond ten days. If you really chew cooked brown rice well, three hundred times or more each mouthful, you begin to understand the meaning of number 7 and George Ohsawa's spirit. Unfortunately, most people didn't do this, and it was years before macrobiotics recovered from the fanatical label that it acquired.

In Boston, we followed developments in New Jersey and New York in sorrow. Afraid that Erewhon would be closed too, we kept the box of Ohsawa's books under Evan's desk. If someone needed a copy, Evan sold them one. TV and radio stations started contacting us. They wanted Michio to appear on the news and defend macrobiotics. He said no. They kept calling and it was hard for us to refuse. A witch-hunt mentality prevailed. We asked Morris Kirsner, our lawyer, to handle it.

Then one day the FBI came to check Erewhon. They really wanted to close us down. Evan was away. Keizo Kushi, Michio's father, was minding the store. He happened to be in Brookline on a visit from Japan. He was a distinguished educator but had trouble understanding spoken English and was slightly deaf. Finally, he called me at home and said some government agents were investigating.

I was in the kitchen cooking. I took off my apron, changed clothes, and rushed right over. The FBI agents were searching the store when I arrived. They wanted to check the back room where the box of *Zen Macrobiotics* books was kept. It was dark. They asked if I had a flashlight. I didn't. They went to their car to get one.

In the few minutes they were gone, I ran into the back room, found the big box of books, and dumped them in a trash can. Then I covered the top with newspapers. When they returned, I escorted them into the back and sat nonchalantly on top of the trash barrel while they searched. Fortunately their flashlight was dim, and they looked in the barrel but didn't find them.

Coming up empty handed, they thanked me politely. Still suspicious, they said they'd like to speak with Michio.

"I'm the sole owner of Erewhon," I told them. "He has nothing to do with the store."

If they had found the books and closed us down, Erewhon might have died in infancy. It was a narrow escape. After that, things relaxed, and natural foods stores were free to sell any books they liked.

The Natural Foods Movement Develops

After the initial furor over macrobiotics died down, our movement progressed unhindered. Until then, there had been a small health food industry in America, carrying mainly wheat germ, brewer's yeast, vitamins, minerals, and other supplements. Macrobiotics favored whole, unprocessed foods, and we didn't want to carry these items. The question came up— how to distinguish macrobiotic stores from ordinary health food stores? In Japanese, we had the term "shizen shoku" or natural foods. I translated directly. Erewhon became known as the Natural Foods Store, and the term spread.

In the beginning, very few natural foods were available, and we brought in traditionally made miso, tamari soy sauce, and other items from abroad. They were expensive and unfamiliar to Americans. However, until good quality food production began in this country, it was necessary to import different items.

As Erewhon started to grow, Paul Hawken, Bill Tara, Neil Rubenstein, Bruce MacDonald, Ron Kotzsch, and other friends came and helped us. Nationally, the organic, whole foods movement began to catch fire. Rachel Carson's bestseller, *Silent Spring*, published the same year as *Zen Macrobiotics*, gave birth to the ecology movement and focused attention on chemical depletion of the soil. Organic farms in New England and elsewhere sprouted up, making good quality seasonal produce available to Erewhon and other natural foods stores.

Organic rice and other grains and beans were still unavailable. Most macrobiotic people still ate River Rice, the commercially grown brown rice from Texas. In California, Chico-San had approached the Lundberg brothers about growing rice without chemicals. They operated a large farm in the Sacramento Valley north of San Francisco. Later, I went out to California to extend my thanks to the Lundbergs for switching to organic methods. I talked about rice as the soul and spirit of culture and civilization in the Far East. I described how it could help improve the health and happiness of modern Western society too.

The Lundberg brothers listened patiently to the tiny Japanese woman in a kimono and asked me how much I was willing to pay for their rice.

I told them, "Rice is priceless. Set a fair price. Whatever it is, we will pay it." A young manager from Erewhon who was accompanying me winced.

The Lundbergs kept their bargain, and we kept ours. Over the years, macrobiotic families around the country have grown up on their pure, nourishing rice. They developed many other organic and naturally made products, ranging from rice cakes to instant foods for traveling. They are true pioneers in the best American tradition.

In Arkansas, Paul Hawken and other Erewhon managers met with Carl Garrich of the Lone Pine Rice and Bean Farm. They made a deal to grow organic brown rice in exchange for guaranteeing their first crop. One by one, farms across the country began to convert to more natural methods. In addition to rice—wheat, barley, oats, rye, and other grains began to be cultivated organically on a commercial scale. Soybeans, azuki beans, lentils, and other beans and legumes that had been grown without chemicals also appeared on natural foods shelves. Sesame seeds and other foods that grew better in other climates were imported by Erewhon. Soon a tremendous variety of wonderful grains, beans, seeds, nuts, and other products from around the world was available relatively inexpensively all around the country.

On Newbury St., Erewhon soon outgrew its original spot and moved into a larger space down the street. But even that proved inadequate to handle increased demand. Warehouse space was leased in South Boston near the waterfront. In addition to distributing whole foods across New England, Erewhon started manufacturing. One of the first products and most popular was peanut butter. Until then, commercially made peanut butter was made in a highly processed way with sugar, additives, and preservatives. At Erewhon we devised a way to make it and preserve the natural taste, flavor, and aroma of the nuts without any sweeteners or artificial ingredients. Natural peanut butter was a big success. The supermarket chains in Boston started carrying it. Erewhon also became widely known for its granolas. Made with sunflower seeds, raisins, nuts, and different natural sweeteners and spices, these attractively boxed cereals offered the first really healthful alternative to highly refined, sugar-frosted breakfast cereals.

The Spiral Widens

As business in the retail store on Newbury Street picked up, my husband needed a larger place to hold his classes. We looked around and rented a room in the Arlington Street Church. A stately Unitarian-Universalist Church adjacent to the Public Gardens, its tall steeple brought back fond memories of my family's church in Yokota. Twice a week, Michio began speaking to all who would listen. There he began to introduce material on the spiral of life, food and human evolution, Oriental healing, the Vega Cycle, ancient and future worlds, natural agriculture, the spiral of history, man/woman relations, biological transmutation, and one peaceful world. Over the years, he would refine and polish these teachings, but they existed in embryo from this time.

The next step was to start a restaurant. Its goal was to introduce delicious natural food to the general public and train future macrobiotic cooks. For nearly a year I searched around for the best place. We finally found a small basement location several blocks from Erewhon. Evan Root served as manager, and Carolyn Heidenry and Peggy Taylor were the first waitresses. We wanted to call it Nowhere, but the city licensing board objected to the name. (Several years later a big seafood restaurant on Boston Wharf opened calling itself No Name and became famous.) I finally picked Sanae, which means "sprouted rice" in Japanese and was Mrs. Ohsawa's name before George renamed her Lima. Later we opened a larger restaurant catercorner from Arlington St. Church and across from the Statler-Hilton. We called it the Seventh Inn, and Mr. Hiroshi Hayashi, a macrobiotic cook from Japan, came over to assume the position of head chef. For years, it was the most elegant macrobiotic restaurant in the country.

Housing the students who started flocking to Boston to study macrobiotics presented a challenge. Many of them were young and hadn't enough money to lease an apartment. Our house had reached the limit of those it could comfortably accommodate. Even as it was, I asked all the boys to cut their hair short in order to blend in with the neighborhood. I started looking all over for another house. Nearby, at 21 University Road, we purchased an apartment with the help of Angela Watson. It enabled many more people to come, live, eat, and study together. We also bought two bicycles, for Paul Hawken and Bill Tara, to commute to work on so they wouldn't have to ride the subway.

Two types of people came to study. The more yang ones, those who were active and social, tended to be more interested in business. They worked at Erewhon, loading and unloading freight, driving trucks, making peanut butter and granola, negotiating with farmers, bankers, and retail store owners. The more yin ones, those who were mental and artistic, tended to be more interested in educational activities. They helped out organizing lectures and seminars and producing our first macrobiotic literature. Jim Ledbetter mimeographed some of Michio's earliest lectures and distributed them under the name of *The Order of the Universe*. Ron Dobrin, Jack Garvey, Rebecca Greenwood, and several other friends put out the first issue of the *East West Journal*. A small 12-page tabloid, it included news of macrobiotic activities around the world, excerpts from my husband's lectures, and recipes and cooking advice from me. Tom Hatch and other friends started Tao Books to publish and distribute macrobiotic literature.

Erewhon West

During the time Erewhon was flourishing on the East Coast,
my youngest son, Hisao, slipped and damaged his knee. He
was about three or four years old and had difficulty walking.
We went to Children's Hospital. The doctors couldn't find
anything wrong. But if he didn't start walking normally again
on his own, they said he would need surgery. My husband
and I were very concerned. From my childhood, I remembered
a special massage used when someone fell down and injured
or damaged their bones in the mountains. Even though a bone
might be crushed to pieces there was a way to clear it up
naturally by just squeezing, stretching, and holding it together.
We called the method *honetsugi*, or bone massage.

We telephoned around. In Los Angeles, I learned of a
Japanese chiropractor who used to use this method for jūdo
practitioners. Instead of having surgery, I took Hisao to
Los Angeles to see this man. We stayed with Jacques De-
Langre in Hollywood. Jacques had studied with the Ohsawas
on their West Coast visits. Later he became known for his
book on *Dō-In*, or self-massage therapy, and for popularizing
traditional, European sourdough bread and different sea salts.
Every day, I would take Hisao by car to Los Angeles' tiny
Japan Town for massage.

I started to think about having natural foods sent to us in
California from Erewhon. Then I thought: why not make
a store here? Chico-San had already started in northern California. There was a growing network of organic farms with
lovely vegetables and fruits. Without telling anyone, I opened
Erewhon-L.A. I rented space near Farmer's Market. Soon
an accountant called me from Erewhon-Boston and told me
I couldn't just go out and open a new store. I told him I was
sorry but I already had.

Bill Tara went to work managing the store. He had begun
teaching macrobiotics and set up a center in Chicago. He had
come out to California to help me drive Hisao to the chiropractor's. For a strong young man, there was not much else

for him to do, and he enjoyed the challenge. As in Boston, Erewhon-L.A. thrived. Later, Bruce MacDonald came, and a warehouse opened. Eventually Tom DeSilva took over the management. It is still doing very well.

The new store naturally attracted students, and I soon needed a place for them to live. In Hollywood, I rented a big house at the corner of Franklin Street, and Bill Tara started giving lectures. The house could accommodate five or six friends besides my other children who came out from Boston to stay with me. After the Franklin Street house filled up, I leased another place, with a big living room and library. It was huge. Thirty people could stay there, and I started making futons for the students to sleep on instead of mattresses. Michio flew out from Boston from time to time to lecture. Many people started macrobiotics there. Meanwhile, Hisao's condition improved. He started to walk normally again. I stayed in Los Angeles two years. Then Carolyn Heidenry came out and took over management of our activities.

Within only a few years, natural foods had spread from coast to coast. Of course, there were many other natural foods companies that developed during these years, including Chico-San, Arrowhead Mills, Westbrae, Eden Foods, and Tree of Life. Among them all, Erewhon earned the reputation as being the pioneer and trendsetter for the whole industry. For the general public, natural peanut butter, granola, and veggie burgers were the introduction to a whole new way of eating. For strict macrobiotic people, these items were eaten more for enjoyment and special occasions. Gradually, good quality, naturally processed, day-to-day foods were introduced such as tofu, *seitan*, tempeh, *natto*, mochi, and sourdough bread.

In the beginning, we had made these foods at home, spending hours in the kitchen cooking the soybeans, kneading the wheat gluten or flour, and pounding the sweet rice. Food made at home like this can never be equalled. As high quality macrobiotic staples became commerically available one by one, for convenience, I began using them at home and in my cooking classes.

But looking back, the early years in Boston and Los Angeles were really special. We had such carefree, happy times together. I remember one morning in Boston, John Polumbo, a student who was staying at our home, asked me to sing five songs, and I danced around the kitchen with a broom. John later started a macrobiotic center in Chicago. The first macrobiotic individuals and families in America passed recipes along from friend to friend, kitchen to kitchen. With no compass to follow but our own intuition, we felt like the ancient Hebrews wandering in the desert or the Puritans sharing the first harvest in Massachusetts Bay. From this tiny seed, our dream of spreading natural foods and realizing one healthy, peaceful world began to take root and flower.

10: East West Teachings and Travels

"A traveler of true means, whatever the day's pace, remembers the provision train." —Lao Tzu

ONE DAY in Brookline, an overseas call came in from Japan. I recognized the voice of a young American friend who had gone to study in Tokyo.

"George Ohsawa has just passed away," he told me.

I couldn't believe it. But he said it was true. I searched a long time in the kitchen and dining room for my husband.

After notifying him, I said, "Michio, I think now you have to study for yourself."

Until then, George Ohsawa had come to visit us once or twice a year. His lectures and talks were enough for us to digest the next six or twelve months. Now we were on our own.

We didn't mourn over Ohsawa's death. There was no sad feeling. He was seventy-two and had led a full, adventurous life. We knew that he would always be with us in spirit.

Later we learned he had died from heart failure. Years before, at Dr. Schweitzer's in Africa, he had deliberately contracted tropical ulcers in an attempt to impress him with macrobiotics. Ohsawa recovered, but afterwards tropical parasites may have remained dormant in his body. Back in Japan, Ohsawa took up his quest again to invent a macrobiotic Coca-Cola. His naturally sweetened herbal beverages were far healthier than ordinary soft drinks. But they may have been too yin for his condition, ultimately reactivating the parasites and weakening his heart.

Despite the shock at his loss, we continued our day-to-day activities. At night when we went to bed, my husband and I realized we couldn't have usual marital relations for a long time. In Japan, there was a saying: "If a close relative passes away, sex is prohibited for forty-nine days." We really understood the meaning of that custom. Out of respect for George Ohsawa's spirit and memory, we abstained naturally, not because we felt we ought to. Then after about a month, when we recovered from our immediate sense of loss, normal relations resumed.

Erewhon had just begun, and Michio had started to teach at the Arlington Street Church. After George Ohsawa passed away, I noticed a tremendous change in my husband. He concentrated all of his energy on teaching his twice weekly lectures, on Tuesdays and Thursdays. He put all his strength into teaching, regardless of who came. Sometimes only one or two students showed up. Undaunted, he would plunge into his subject. He never canceled a lecture or waited for more students to arrive. Michio always went straight ahead, like an arrow. With Ohsawa now gone, the future of macrobiotics lay squarely on his shoulders.

In the beginning, Michio was rather weak. As a university student, he had some symptoms of tuberculosis. They had cleared up when food shortages and rationing during the war forced everyone to eat simply and chew well. In Hiyoshi, Michio had studied a total of only about 48 hours with George Ohsawa. He would commute from his international law studies at Tokyo University and spend a few hours at the Maison Ignoramus discussing world affairs. George Ohsawa recognized Michio's brilliant mind and universal spirit. He hoped that his young visitor would someday discover food as the key to world health and world peace.

When he came to America, Michio was not really following a macrobiotic way of eating. If I have succeeded at all as his partner in life, it is in seeing to his day-to-day nourishment. On visits to America, George Ohsawa treated Michio more as an associate than as a student. In turn, Michio very much respected Ohsawa. But he did not regard him as his superior in the way I did. Our different views came to a head the morning of the Ohsawas' arrival in New York. I had been so eager to see them. For days I had talked of nothing else.

On the way to the Buddhist temple, Michio and I got into an argument in the car. "Don't say, 'George, George, George,' all the time," he said. "I'm going to go my own way."

I was in a hurry to get there and driving very fast. "Oh my gosh, how will he behave to George?" I thought. I kept still and eased up on the accelerator. But when we got there, Michio was his usual smiling, polite self. The two men talked very warmly together, without hesitation. I noticed only that they didn't bow in the Japanese fashion. I knew that George Ohsawa didn't care for formalities any more than Michio. Everything went smoothly. I was relieved.

Over the years, George Ohsawa acquired a reputation for scolding his students. In Japan, I faced his scorn many times. In New York, though he attacked many other macrobiotic friends, George never scolded Michio. In Cambridge, George's paternal affection continued. When he was accused in the acupuncture case, my husband received a telegram from George in France: "Congratulations, Michio, you have now become an adult."

But finally one time George wrote Michio accusing him of something in a two-page letter. Michio was upset. It was the first time he had faced Papa's wrath. In anger, he tore up the letter. I found the scraps and pieced them together again with Scotch tape.

"This is very reasonable," I told my husband after reading the letter.

Michio quickly got over his impatience. It was the first and only attack he received.

George Ohsawa's behavior toward Michio illustrated the antagonistic side to his character. Throughout his life, George had strongly attacked other people in his letters and magazines. In person, he was very gentle, humorous, and understanding. He was almost unable to criticize anyone to their face. When people later received his hammer blow in print, they felt betrayed. Many people couldn't understand this behavior and left him.

Later, we understood that this was a manifestation of Ohsawa's native constitution. He was born October 17. People born in the fall and winter are generally mentally and emotionally inclined. Outwardly, George was very passionate and aggressive, but when he attacked someone, it was usually at a distance. Lima was just the opposite. She was born in April. People born in the spring and summer have a more yang constitution. They are more physical and social. Outwardly, they are often gentle and meek, but inwardly they are very strong. At the Maison Ignoramus, it was always frail Lima who would deliver the bad news in person.

Michio was also born in the spring, on May 17. Many revolutionists have been born in mid-May. Naturally, Michio and George's experience and way of teaching were completely different. Though somewhat the same, their original constitution created the difference. Overall, they were going in the same direction, even if they developed their own way. George's and Michio's families originated only about a half hour away from each other in Kumano, a beautiful area of Japan noted for the natural beauty of its land and ocean and the spiritual depth of its people.

George really depended on Michio and had great hopes for him. Their meeting, though by chance, was the result of past karma. After George Ohsawa passed away, my husband fully developed himself. He devoted himself tirelessly to reconstructing modern society and turning the world away from biological degeneration and the threat of war. As his partner, I unconditionally supported him in realizing his dream.

Macrobiotic Education

Macrobiotics in the United States spread in a spiral. The first young people to study with us came from San Francisco and the West Coast. Some of them were very yin, primarily hippies seeking a "natural high" or instant *satori*—a taste of enlightenment. The next circle was smaller. Many friends came from Minnesota such as Bill Gleason, Tom Hatch, and Leonard and Barbara Jacobs. Ken Burns came from Detroit. Like Midwesterners in general, they were very yang. They excelled in business and other practical pursuits. The third wave came from an even shorter distance: New York, Pennsylvania, and Connecticut. They included Denny Waxman, Murray Snyder, Edward and Wendy Esko, and Sherman Goldman. They tended to be more moderate, balancing an interest in art and spiritual development with business and teaching.

By the early 1970s, Boston had become the hub of macrobiotic activities nationwide. Erewhon had grown into a multimillion dollar business, manufacturing and distributing natural foods from coast to coast. Following the example of Erewhon, thousands of natural foods stores, coops, and restaurants had opened, many by students who had come to study with us or with the handful of macrobiotic teachers in New York or California.

In Boston itself, Erewhon now had three retail stores in addition to the warehouse. Hundreds of people worked for the company. Orders that came into the Watts lines in the morning were loaded onto big tractor-trailer trucks in the afternoon. Special railroad cars containing organically grown wheat, rice, sesame seeds, and other products came in to nearby South Station, Boston's central rail terminal. In the warehouse, the food would be weighed, sifted, made into whole grain flour or otherwise processed and then be put into 100-, 50-, or 25-pound sacks for delivery to retail stores.

In Japan, we made arrangements with friends to set up a new macrobiotic distribution company. It was named Mitoku and was selected from the initial letters of our names in Japanese: *Mi*chio and *To*moko *Ku*shi. Over the years, Mitoku and Muso, another macrobiotic food company based in Osaka, introduced hundreds of high quality products. Like Erewhon and Chico-San in America, they sought out and encouraged the few remaining organic farmers, traditional miso-makers, tea bush growers, seaweed cultivators, and other small natural foods manufacturers in Japan. Though not so well known, Mr. Akiyoshi Kazama, the owner of Mitoku, is responsible for the development of many of these products and the improved health of thousands of families in America, Japan, and around the world. We are very grateful for his services and always look forward to visiting him and his gracious wife on our visits to Tokyo.

In Boston our study houses grew apace of Erewhon and Mitoku's flourishing activity. At their peak, we had ten houses in all, including three in Brookline, two in Cambridge, two in Alston, and one in Newton. There, friends working at Erewhon, the two restaurants, and the *East West Journal* could live in a harmonious environment, receive well balanced meals, and study macrobiotics. In Ashburnham, about an hour northwest of Boston, we purchased land and started to develop a rural community. Friends who wanted to live in the woods, meditate, or experiment with natural building or agriculture found an opportunity there, though the community in Ashburnham as a whole never really developed.

Once good quality natural foods had become established, we could turn our attention to education. In Japan, teaching had been my profession. Michio also had a background in the field. Both of his parents were educators, and he had taught at a Catholic girls' high school before coming to the United States. Both of us enjoyed teaching and were greatly influenced by our senior teachers. In my husband's case, this included not only George Ohsawa, but also Professor Shigeru Nanbara, Chancellor of Tokyo University; Professor Toyohiko Hori, a law professor and Christian; and Rev. Toyohiko Kagawa, a Christian theologian and international peace promoter. When he first came to America, Michio went to see many great men in his quest for a way to lasting peace including Albert Einstein, Thomas Mann, Upton Sinclair, Norman Cousins, Pitirim Sorokin, and Robert M. Hutchins. He always regarded them as respected elders.

Our life together was destined to center on education. We did not really study education as a system or learn all the formal techniques of teaching. But even during the early years in New York, struggling to survive, we had no doubt that a way would develop for us to realize our dream.

From the macrobiotic perspective, nature and the universe are our ultimate teachers. Daily life offers lessons that cannot be learned in any classroom. Living together as a family, or with other people, involves constant learning. Many forms of education automatically established themselves after moving to Boston. Our system of study houses developed very naturally among people who came to study with us. The small, informal family-style accommodations we set up enabled hundreds of people to study basic macrobiotics. The experienced guided the inexperienced. As their health and judgment improved, newer people moved up into positions of responsibility. Older people who had been with us a few years went back to their homes or out into the world to set up their own centers. In this way, people constantly spiralled in and out of Boston.

To set up schools required teachers, administration, and finances—all of which we lacked. In the beginning, we prided ourselves on having no entrance examinations and no degrees. Ours was a School of Life. Supreme judgment reigned. The Order of the Universe governed all of our actions. Health and happiness, or sickness and sorrow, were entirely up to every individual. Each of us possessed the key to infinite realization. By eating and chewing well, we controlled our own destiny. Once Ty Smith, who became head of Erewhon, compared our educational movement to the yoga movement and other alternative lifestyles. He described macrobiotics in Boston as the "communityless community."

Our community grew naturally in the way a seedling develops into a tree, putting down roots and spreading out branches. Gradually our activities expanded. Our students started their own natural foods companies, teaching centers, and business enterprises. The men gave dietary and way of life consultations. The ladies gave cooking classes. Others went into organic farming and gardening or made natural clothing, bedding, and cosmetics. In our view, all of these activities were interrelated and part of macrobiotic education.

Usually in the evening, after work, friends gathered for Michio's lectures. His talks expanded from two nights a week to five. Before long, there were activities on the weekends. Regular attendance grew from a handful of students to dozens, from dozens to fifty or one hundred and more. On special occasions, such as a symposium or a natural foods expo, thousands of people would gather to hear this skinny Japanese man in a three-piece suit talk about brown rice and miso soup as the key to health, peace, and spiritual development.

As macrobiotics grew, we set up the East West Foundation for public education and rented space in the building next to the Arlington Street Church on Boylston Street. My children were now all in school, and I could devote more time to teaching. In addition to cooking, I gave classes in the Tea Ceremony, flower arrangement, and futon making. I also brought to Boston a Noh drama master whom I had studied with in Los Angeles. In Boston, our cultural activities became as well known as our dietary and health-related activities. My husband and I dined with Edwin O. Reischaeur, the former American ambassador to Japan, and his lovely Japanese wife at the Seventh Inn. We asked him what had changed the most in Japan. He immediately replied, "Japanese women." The *East West Journal* became the voice of the emerging New Age movement, distributing tens of thousands of copies around the country each month.

World Travels

From Europe, South America, Canada, and other countries, many friends came to study with us in Boston. Ferro Ledvinka came from Italy, Richard Theobald from Germany, Marc Van Cauwenberghe, a young medical doctor, from Belgium, and dozens of Flemish people. Afterwards they went home to introduce macrobiotics and set up centers. Soon we received invitations to travel abroad and teach.

For many years, we had not been able to travel out of the
United States because of our immigration problems. In New
York, we had finally received a business visa in connection
with our import-export activities. However, after moving to
Cambridge, we sold those businesses and received another
deportation notice. Our lawyer, Morris Kirsner, referred us to
an immigration lawyer, and we applied for permanent resident
status. When George Ohsawa died, we wanted to travel to
Japan and pay our respects. But we were in the middle of this
case and were afraid we wouldn't be let back in the country.
A few years later, our immigration problems were resolved.
We were free to travel out of the country. As world citizens,
we felt the whole concept of modern states and nations was
obsolete.

Our first trip was to Europe. A doctor invited us to teach
in London. Bill Tara was there then. He had gone to India
enroute to Japan to join Paul Hawken, Evan Root, and several
other Erewhon managers. On the way home, he came back
via England, where he stayed and set up the Community
Health Foundation. Our first lecture was held in London in
the Tara Hotel near Hyde Park. When I first met Bill Tara
in Boston, I remember laughing at his name. In Japanese,
tara means codfish. In London I was surprised at the name of
the hotel. I learned that it was a very old name. Many Irish
kings were named Tara.

My husband spoke for five days, in the mornings and afternoons. Many doctors, health professionals, and friends attended. They came from all around England as well as Belgium
and Holland. Michio's talks were recorded, and Bill said they
amounted to over ten miles of tape. From London we went to
Paris. Karin Stephan, a lovely young macrobiotic yoga teacher,
and Jean Bernard Rishi, whose daughter later married our son,
arranged a seminar for us. We stayed near the UNESCO
headquarters. Many friends gathered. It was the first macrobiotic seminar in Paris since George Ohsawa had passed away,
and it was our first visit to France since 1952.

George Ohsawa especially loved Paris. He had lived there

in the early 1930s and again in the mid-1950s and early 1960s. He was particularly fond of the *marronnier* or horse-chestnut. He described it vividly in his lectures. In my mind, I confused it with macaroni, which had a similar pronunciation. In my diary years ago at the M.I. I had written, "I would like to go to Paris where the 'macaroni' flowers blossom." George laughed and laughed. The sight of that flowering tree brought back happy memories of my days in Hiyoshi.

In Paris, we attended a banquet in memory of Ohsawa. Some Japanese macrobiotic friends strung up a banner:

> George Ohsawa passed away and was buried in Japan,
> But his soul is still alive in Paris.

We met Clim Yoshimi, who served as Ohsawa's secretary and French translator, and Abe Nakamura, my old classmate at the Maison Ignoramus who helped me get my visa to America. He and Aida, his pretty wife, had moved to Germany and were teaching macrobiotics in Dusseldorf.

Since our first trip to Europe, we have returned about two or three times a year to give seminars and cooking classes. We also started traveling to Central and South America and the Far East, visiting altogether dozens of countries. I have learned many things on my travels and would like to share some of my impressions.

England

I have visited Great Britain many times. Even though my English is funny, I can go around by myself to see places. I enjoy London. It is a big international city with wide thoroughfares and spacious parks. I also like visiting the countryside. The traditional thatched-roof houses are very small but homey. They remind me of farmers' dwellings in Japan. In college, I read many books in English literature. I loved Dickens, especially *The Tale of Two Cities*, the poetry of Byron and Shelley, Conan Doyle's Sherlock Holmes stories, and Agatha Christie's mysteries. Traveling through England,

I always think of these authors and their wonderful creations. I also saw many historical sites, including Stonehenge and some ancient castles. One time I saw the Tower of London. It produced in me very strange feelings.

Over the years many people came to study with us in London. But since Bill Tara was organizing our seminars, we didn't deal directly with many English friends. In general, I found the British proud, very well mannered, and sincere. Our first European Macrobiotic Congress, with delegates from many countries in Europe, was held in London. Lima Ohsawa came from Japan as honorary president, and we have happy memories of that gathering.

Belgium

When I was selling George Ohsawa's World Government newspaper in Tokyo, one of the first world citizens' congresses was held in Geneva and Paris. In Belgium, Pière Gaveart was also promoting that assembly. His father, Edgar, had escaped to England during the war and was very active in world peace activities. The Gavearts started corresponding with Ohsawa in Tokyo. After leaving Africa, the Ohsawas visited Belgium and helped the Gavearts set up the first macrobiotic food company in Europe. They named it Lima in honor of Mrs. Ohsawa. Michio and I had long known about the Gavearts but had never met them. Then after fifteen years had passed, we finally met Pière, his wife, and their wonderful mother in Ghent. We were just like brothers and sisters who had not seen each other for ages. It was wonderful.

Our seminars in Belgium were usually held in Ghent or Antwerp. Each city was traditional but rather dark. During both World War I and II, Belgium was at the crossroads of the battlefields. I found the Belgium and Flemish people themselves flexible, strong, and unified. I was continually impressed at the way they always helped each other. Whenever we wanted to bring people in Europe together, we could always count on our friends in Belgium to organize things.

The Netherlands

Amsterdam, the main city in Holland, is very active and dynamic. Beginning in about the fourteenth to sixteenth centuries, the Dutch people were very active throughout the world. They settled Manhattan Island in New York and established colonies in the East and West Indies. After visiting Holland, I could understand the source of their power. The energy in Holland is very floating, water-type energy. It is constantly in motion, flowing, melting, swirling, shaping. Over the years we have held many seminars in Amsterdam. Adelbert and Wieke Nelissen, our hosts, have been very active in macrobiotic food distribution and education, establishing Manna Foods, publishing books, and teaching throughout Europe.

France

George Ohsawa first started teaching macrobiotics in France over fifty years ago. Many persons have benefited. But over the years, the macrobiotic community has never been able to unite. The French are very individualistic. Ten to fifteen times, we gave seminars in France, but the leaders, organizers, and centers always changed. There was no continuity. Instead of helping each other, people appeared to be discouraging each other. Yet as individuals, the French are very beautiful and gifted. It is truly amazing to watch. Sometimes I wished to organize them.

I asked myself what accounts for this paradox? I finally realized the French are just like grapes. While some foods like apples are one, grapes are divided. There are many grapes to each cluster.

"The French people have a grape mentality," I mentioned one time.

My friend Hélène Magalino replied, "Yes, but when an emergency comes, they come together. In a crisis, they make the best wine."

It is true. During World War II, the French united to form the Resistance to Nazi brutality. However, most of the time the French like to avoid being crushed and display their individualistic flavors and tastes. I have come to enjoy each friend from France very much.

Switzerland

Switzerland's natural beauty and cleanliness make it an ideal place to teach macrobiotics. The mountains are beautiful, the valleys serene. Almost every corner of the country is well taken care of. Our first seminar in Switzerland was in Gestaad. Madame Toutier organized it, and we enjoyed it very much. In the Alps, we conducted seminars at a yearly summer camp. One year in Lenk, several hundred people from twenty-three countries came. Michio's lectures were simultaneously translated into five languages. Every July we continue to attend this gathering. The Swiss have a long history of international service, neutrality, and peace promotion. In recent years, our associates, including Mario Binetti, Katriona Forrester, and others, set up one of the Kushi Institutes in Kiental, a beautiful Swiss mountain community.

Germany

I went to the Black Forest of southern Germany for one seminar. The soil was very rich, as in Austria where we had lectured in Innsbruck. Many famous musicians were born in this part of Germany. I could feel the music naturally arising from the land itself. We also taught in Frankfurt, Bonn, and Munich. Central Germany is an amazing industrial area, especially along the Alsatian border where Dr. Schweitzer came from. I felt so sorry for this area because of the pollution.

As a whole, Germany produced in me a deep, rich feeling. The German people are very steady, dependable, and orderly. We found German young people trying to escape the authoritarianism of the past. In macrobiotics, they see a happy,

healthy alternative to the horrors of the Second World War
and the Cold War that have divided their nation. There are
heavy tensions, and I understand there is a big fence between
East and West Berlin.

In Japan, people have mostly forgotten the difficult days of
the war. They have admitted the mistakes of the past and
moved on. In Germany, the agony of the war still continues.
One of the differences may be the nature of the fighting.
Hiroshima and Nagasaki were destroyed by atomic bombs.
People there suffered terrible fates, as did those in Tokyo
during the fire-bombings. However, in daily life, the Japanese
people didn't face an enemy they could see.

In Europe, the war pitted country against country, culture
against culture, neighbor against neighbor. Terrible things
were done on a personal scale. Feelings and memories ran
much deeper. In Germany we were surprised that people
didn't discuss the holocaust.

In the Far East, bloody wars had also occurred from time
to time in the past. In Japan, for example, many Christians
were massacred in the early seventeenth century when the
Tokugawa era began. When such cruel things happened,
people traditionally built a shrine or temple in memory of
their families or ancestors. Even a small shrine or altar in the
home can help the spirits of those who have died make a
smooth transition to the next world. For the living, a shrine
can also help create a peaceful vibration in a place where violence and bloodshed have occurred.

To recover its health and begin to move in a harmonious
direction, Germany will have to let go of the modern diet.
Sausage, wurst, hard salted cheese, and other animal foods
create a tremendous attachment to the past. In combination
with excessive pastries, refined flour, beer, and other extreme
yin items, these foods will lead to continuing imbalance,
including fear, defensiveness, and guilt. Narrow, rigid ways
of thinking and acting will begin to melt naturally when
people start returning to a more balanced way of eating. In
Germany we came to love traditional pumpernickel bread,

naturally fermented sauerkraut, and delicious dishes made with wheat, oats, rye, millet, and other whole grains that have been cultivated for centuries. Once Germany establishes strong macrobiotic practice and cooking, it will greatly influence other countries as in the past.

Denmark

I knew Denmark from reading Hans Christian Andersen's stories as a child. Copenhagen, the capital, is a beautiful place and the people are plain and friendly. There are no signs or billboards, as in Vermont. We were very impressed. In college I loved reading Ibsen and felt close to the Scandinavian people. Someday I would like to visit Sweden and Norway.

Eastern Europe and Russia

I have not been to Yugoslavia but have met many people from there. From childhood, I loved Russian and Slavic folk songs and movies. In college a favorite was "The Song of the Flower." The music seemed to come from the center of the earth. Lino Stanchich, now a senior macrobiotic teacher in the United States, came from Yugoslavia. He has a very strong constitution. Recently, several other Yugoslavians have studied with us in Boston. Their voices also naturally came from the *hara*, the energy center deep in the intestines. I could feel their strength. No one can compete with the native constitutions of our friends from Yugoslavia and other Eastern European countries.

Macrobiotic activities have begun in Yugoslavia, Rumania, Hungary, Poland, Czechoslovakia, and other parts of Eastern Europe. It is only a matter of time before they reach the Soviet Union. Natural foods can cross international borders very easily. As our way of life spreads, health, harmony, and peace will naturally follow.

Italy

We have visited Italy many times, giving seminars in Rome, Milan, and Florence. My favorite place is Florence. I can walk around the city all day and never get tired. I also enjoy Assisi, visiting the ancient town where St. Francis lived. South Italy is very different from North Italy. Once we went to Sicily. It had the best spaghetti we had ever tasted. Usually we have difficulty eating when we travel. In many countries natural foods, fresh produce, or foods cooked without sugar and chemicals are hard to find. Japan is the worst place to travel if you are macrobiotic. Italy is the best. If we carry our own tamari soy sauce and condiments, we enjoy Italian noodles and pasta very much. Also, in Italy people still eat together as a family. This makes for strong family unity.

The Italian people themselves are very active. They are not so individualistic as the French or as group-oriented as the Germans. They are artistic, gay, and warm. Though I don't speak Italian, I love to listen to it. It is such a happy language. Italian has a musical quality that people who speak English appreciate. Perhaps this is one reason so many of Shakespeare's plays are set in this lovely country.

Spain

The people of Spain are very different from Italians. They are more passionate, aggressive, and devout. Catholic traditions are much stronger there than anywhere else we visited in Europe. We have taught in Madrid and Barcelona many times. Macrobiotic friends took us to a very good seafood restaurant. We had *paella* with seafood and enjoyed it very much. It reminded me exactly of Mother's *gomoku* rice which she made for Christmas holy day.

Often our seminars in Spain would be held in old cathedrals or churches. We also very much enjoy the Basque country. It has so many beautiful flowers. Once Tony Sattilaro, a doctor who had overcome cancer with the help of macrobiotics, came with us. Our hosts presented Michio and Dr. Satillaro traditional Basque black hats after the seminar. Their names were embroidered around the headbands. Later we went on to Portugal. On the way, we remembered that it was Michio's birthday. We had completely forgotten. Usually we are too busy to celebrate our birthdays at home. I was pleased that our Basque friends knew intuitively and gave my husband a present.

Portugal

Portugal holds a special place in my heart. In the countryside, the people remind me very much of people in rural Japan. The older villagers look, talk, and act just like Japanese farmers and fishermen. The expression on their faces is exactly the same. I think this comes from eating mostly grains and vegetables and fish and seafood. In Portugal, it is also relatively easy to eat well while traveling. The food is simple and wholesome. We enjoy the fish and seafood, especially rice paella and *calamari* and squid. *Castella* (couscous cakes) are also very delicious.

Michio usually doesn't have time to sight-see. But in Portugal, there is an old castle in Cintra, just outside of Lisbon, that he likes to visit. It dates back to medieval times. After Marco Polo and other travelers visited the Far East, some adventurous Orientals came West. About four or five hundred years ago, a small delegation of Japanese samurai was sent to Rome to train as Catholic priests. They were very young, only in their teens. They traveled by a Portuguese ship and stopped and visited this castle. In Rome, they went to many Catholic churches. But while they were in Italy, a new shōgun came to power in Japan. He changed policy. Christianity was prohibited and went underground. For the next three hundred years, Japan's door to the West remained closed. The samurai came back home unable to complete their training. But they may not have returned empty-handed. They may have brought back to Japan the art of cooking *tempura*, which originated in Portugal.

Outside of Lisbon, near another famous castle, is Linho

prison. One time, Chico Varatojo, a dynamic young man who studied with us in Boston, took us out there. He had set up a center in Lisbon and was going out several times a week to teach macrobiotics at the maximum-security penitentiary. It was the first time I had ever visited a prison, and I was a little apprehensive. I thought we would say hello to everyone and come right back.

My fears were groundless. It was a wonderful, enlightening experience. We stayed until visiting hours ended, over three hours. Everyone was waiting for us in a large room where they ate together. They were not allowed to use knives but somehow they managed to cut the vegetables. The young men were very sincere and eager to learn. They asked us wonderful questions. Usually people ask us about their physical condition. Even longtime students are always asking our advice on how to ease some minor ache or pain. But these friends asked us about philosophical and social questions. We were very impressed. My husband and I felt we had at last found a group of real macrobiotic revolutionaries.

After my visit to Linho, I felt I understood the meaning of *Erewhon* for the first time. In his satire, Samuel Butler suggested that criminals be put in the hospital, while sick people should be put in jail. In the Erewhonian hospitals, offenders were given proper food and quickly recovered their health and judgment. Crime was seen as a biochemical imbalance. As in Linho, criminals in the land of Erewhon were often the most active, adventurous, and naive persons. In contrast, those who did not observe natural law became sick. In the eyes of the Order of the Universe, sickness was a heavier crime. The sick were punished for not taking responsibility for their health and happiness.

Later, most of the men in Linho eating macrobiotically were released early. The authorities recognized their changed attitude and behavior but thought it was due to their belief, not to the food itself. One former prisoner, Antonio "Toze" Aréal, came to study with us in Boston. In his youth, he had become heavily involved in narcotics, weaponry, and terrorism.

In prison, he was known as one of the most dangerous men in Portugal. But when he came out, he was completely changed thanks to macrobiotics. In Brookline, he lived at our home and often helped me cook dinner in the kitchen. Everyone was deeply impressed with his earnest attitude and shy, gentle demeanor. On Cape Cod, he helped set up a macrobiotic center in Portuguese-speaking New Bedford. Now back in Portugal, he is actively teaching and is married and has a family.

Someday prisons and hospitals as we know them will become a thing of the past. Health care and correctional centers around the world will serve high-quality natural foods. People with physical or psychological disorders, as well as those with unfocused surplus energy, will go there. After a short period of good food, proper exercise, self-reflection, and studies in natural order, they will be well enough to rejoin society.

The Middle East

I grew up to stories of Moses crossing the Red Sea and entering the Holy Land. I especially liked the psalms of David and memorized many of them. I thought Palestine and Israel must be very beautiful, flowing with milk and honey. The first time I saw a movie in New York about the Middle East, I was shocked. It was mostly desert with so many stones. It didn't match my creative imagination. Jerusalem, of course, was different. I knew the Temple was ruined. We have many macrobiotic friends in Lebanon, Israel, Saudi Arabia, and other Middle Eastern countries. They are working for peace amidst so much fear and violence. Someday my husband and I hope to visit macrobiotic centers in this part of the world and teach.

Central and Latin America

We visited Costa Rica many times. It is a beautiful country and very unique because it has no army. Michio spoke at a world government convention and gave dietary and way of life consultations to the president and former president of Costa Rica. We also went to Venezuela and enjoyed the islands and high mountains. In Caracas, there is much pollution, and I felt sorry for the people. Once I went to Brazil and traveled along the beautiful coastline from Rio to São Paulo. It was the first time I crossed the equator. Physically it was a very long trip. My mind couldn't adjust. I felt like I was seeing my back. I realized traveling from East to West was much easier than North to South. I found macrobiotic people in Central and Latin America very active. friendly, and earnest. They were not so conceptual. I enjoyed talking with them directly heart to heart.

I have not yet seen the Andes Mountains and someday hope to visit Peru. In Central and Latin America, I sampled many beautiful corn dishes. The first time I tasted *arepas* cooked with whole corn it opened my mind to the possibility of making delicious, nourishing corn dishes without cornmeal. Machecha, a lovely woman from Venezuela who lives in Boston and has studied with us, has taught many macrobiotic friends how to prepare whole corn in the traditional way.

North America

My travels helped me see the United States in better perspective. Compared to Europeans, Americans are less intellectual and philosophical. Europeans understand macrobiotic theory more deeply. They have a long, rich cultural background and identify strongly with the land where they were born. However, their understanding tends to be conceptual, and sometimes their practice is tight or shallow. Americans are more practical. They are idealistic but not ideological. Their understanding is flexible and adaptable, and their practice is generally well balanced. Americans also are more cooperative than Europeans. I think this comes about because the United States is more spread out. Americans can embrace many different cultures. There is more space, more synthesis, more appreciation of the whole. Europeans have been living in small well-defined territories for centuries. As food changes from one region to another, the culture changes. There is less mingling than in America. The United States does not have a set cultural structure. Though it is the worldwide leader of modern civilization, overall America is less rigid than most other countries.

On my travels, I have come to see that the differences between people are greatly influenced by the atmospheric energy, geographical location, weather, and climate, as well as by food. Generally, people living in regions or countries to the North are steadier, quieter, and less expressive than people to the South. People in the south are happier, more animated, and more relaxed. They even smile more. In the United States, I enjoy the South very much. Over the years, we have given many seminars in Miami, Atlanta, Dallas, and Houston. I especially like the mountains of South Carolina. The air there is more humid. It feels very much like central Japan. New England's climate is more like Hokkaido, the cold, northern island of Japan.

The Far East

Because of modern artificial development, nature around the world now is being destroyed. Everywhere people are unhappy. Wars and conflicts are spreading. I used to take comfort in the fact that the land survived. As an old poem said:

> The country is defeated,
> But the mountains and rivers still live on.

Today, the mountains and rivers are dying, although the world as a whole is not at war. This is especially true in Japan. The land there is being destroyed by the prosperity of modern civilization, not by fighting. In Japan, macrobiotics is difficult to spread because people are seeking everything Western. Our expression is still too Japanese for them.

Present day Japan is not the traditional Orient. That exists now only in our memory. One of the biggest differences between Japan and America is the number of lawyers in this country. My husband and I noticed this from the beginning. Almost everyone has a lawyer. People use the law to their own advantage, accusing others, defending themselves, seeking advantage. They think nothing of suing someone else. Even marriage has become a legal contract, with husband and wife protecting their material wealth from each other. Family unity, community harmony, and world peace are very difficult to achieve when such mistrust prevails.

Growing up, I never saw a lawyer. In our valley, there was only one. He registered real estate, and his job paid poorly. We never had any "No Trespassing" signs in Izumo province. Of course, shrines, temples, and other special places were protected by custom. But we could go anywhere in the countryside, in the mountains, or along the beach. There were no restrictions, no "Keep Out" signs as in the United States. In present-day Japan, the number of lawyers is on the increase

People in East and West are not really different at all. The difference is between traditional and modern society. People in an agricultural society eat mainly grains and vegetables. They are very friendly, sharing and cooperating with one another. They see things from many points of view. They look at themselves as custodians of the land, not as owners. People in modern industrial society eat mostly meat, sugar, dairy food, refined flour and grains, canned food, and other highly processed items. They become very possessive. They see things only from their own perspective. They look at the land as private property for their own personal enjoyment. This is a big source of unhappiness in the world today.

After coming to the United States, my husband and I did not go back to Japan for over twenty years. Our Japanese friends who visited America and our American friends who came back from trips to Japan kept us informed about radical changes there. In 1971, after our visa problems were settled, we went back for the first time. We really felt like Rip Van Winkles. There were so many changes. The Tokyo skyline was completely rebuilt and looked like big international cities everywhere. But some things had remained the same. The exit of Tokyo Station where I sold George Ohsawa's World Government newspaper was still boarded up.

In Tokyo, we saw Lima and other macrobiotic friends. After George died, Lima had a difficult time. She was not outgoing or social. She was more of a traditional Japanese wife, keeping the home beautiful and taking care of her husband and family. She had no desire to lead. But with George gone, she was pushed into the forefront of macrobiotic activities. She devoted herself to teaching cooking and set up the Nippon C.I. in a small western suburb of Tokyo. C.I. stood for Center Ignoramus. The name came from the old M.I., Maison Ignoramus, in Hiyoshi. Lima was beautifully attired as usual. She wore long, graceful dresses or soft skirts and ruffled blouses in the French style. Her hair was done up in an elegant bouffant. She looked radiant and younger than her actual age. She welcomed us warmly. As always, we felt elevated by her modest and humble spirit. Many people from around the world studied with her after her husband passed away. She has had a wonderful influence, sowing seeds of health and happiness wherever she goes.

In Izumo province, I had another warm reunion. I went to see Mr. Tanaka, my teacher in college. I had not been in touch with him since leaving Japan. He was glad to see me and thanked me for the ball-point pen I sent twenty years earlier. Shortly after arriving in the United States, I had given someone coming back to Japan a small package to deliver to him. There was only my M.I. name, Asta, on it. Mr. Tanaka recognized it at once. Since I had put no address on the parcel, he could not reach me.

In Yokota, I visited my family, and in Maki I visited my former elementary school students. In New York and Boston, I often thought of my days in the mountains, teaching eager, bright-eyed country girls. I had only to close my eyes and vivid images would come to my mind. I could see rice ears ripening in the fields, clear peaks etched in the autumn sky, and cold springs issuing from rocks that we picked up in our hands after pushing aside the fallen leaves. My former students were now married with families of their own. We had a lovely time reminiscing.

I decided to publish a small book of haiku my students had written in class during the war. Over the years, I had read them many times. Their freshness and originality moved me more deeply than the poems of Basho and other great haiku masters. I asked Mr. Tanaka to write the foreword. In a beautiful introduction, he described our friendship over the years. He observed my changing image clearly. He noted how my personality had deepened as I went from being a student to a teacher and how I had been affected by my sickness and studying with George Ohsawa.

> I think Miss Yokoyama's gifts are heaven-sent, and she has developed them as intended. But until then, there was an internal spiritual struggle and the pain of sickness. Through these difficulties, the foundation of her personality was built. She went on to study with Mr. Sakurazawa and married Mr. Kushi. Both made her a great woman, I guess.
>
> This collection of poems is not only interesting as an anthology but also lets us feel the true heart of humanity. Her radiance and personality shine through, making this book of poems true.

My husband also contributed to the book's opening pages. He wrote a poem contrasting the children's simple, clear natural way of life with the chaos of the Second World War.

> In the midst of a series of insane battles,
> Human life rises and falls,
> Flourishes and dies.
> The stars come out,
> The spring haze appears.
> The songs of the young children of Maki

Strain the heart,
Echoing ripples in the mountain streams,
Reflecting white clouds floating in the sky.

Except for Japan, and brief visits to Hong Kong, I haven't
traveled in Asia. I would like to visit China, India, Malaysia,
and many other countries. Our students have begun to spread
macrobiotic teachings in these regions. There are also macrobiotic activities in Australia, and maybe one day we will
journey there. Each country has a traditional culture and
cuisine awaiting to be rediscovered. The future world of health
and happiness will be a harmonious mosaic of teachings,
musical and artistic approaches, and balanced ways of eating
drawn from many lands.

Africa

My husband and I visited Africa for the first time in 1987.
We had been invited to the Congo by government health
officials to give a conference and public lecture on the macrobiotic approach to AIDS. Our meetings were held at W.H.O.
regional headquarters in Brazzaville, the capital, and two
hundred African medical doctors attended.

In July, during African winter, the weather is mild. It was
cooler than Boston. I was so surprised. During our stay, we
toured the outlying savannah and met many villagers. In the
countryside, the people follow a more traditional way of
eating and are generally in good health. We visited a convent
where the sisters have an organic garden and are interested
in learning how to make tofu and tempeh. Both Michio and
I were impressed with the Africans' physical beauty, graceful
movement, and calm, gentle nature. The women wore beautiful clothing and carried big jars on their head.

Water is a major problem. During the dry season, people
walk miles to fetch water for daily cooking and cleaning.
To wash I learned to dip a corner of a small cloth in the
bucket and use it to moisten my face and hands. Despite

such hardships, the people are grateful for the little they have
and keep a bright, cheerful mind.

In the cities, the traditional way of eating is no longer
observed. Following colonialism and international relief
shipments, sugar, dairy food, refined flour, and canned food
have replaced whole grains and other staples. The result is
increased illness including AIDS and other diseases of modern
civilization.

Our trip was arranged by Henri and Hélène Lucy, a couple
of French descent who head a big construction company in
Brazzaville. Several years ago, Hélène had pancreatic cancer
and recovered after a year of careful eating in Becket. Since
then, she and her husband have devoted themselves whole-
heartedly to spreading macrobiotics, setting up Kushi
Institutes in France and the Congo.

Thanks to the Lucys' efforts, along with a delegation of
macrobiotic cooks, teachers, and medical friends which accompanied us together with many African scientists, doctors, and
nutritionists, the conference was a big success. The Congo
government asked us to begin macrobiotic education in
clinics, hospitals, and schools. Upon our return to America,
many young macrobiotic friends, especially those who speak
French, volunteered to go to Africa to teach cooking, farming,
miso making, and other skills. We often say a peaceful mind
depends on a healthy body. In the same way, without healthy
land, a peaceful society will never come. Restoring agriculture
and attending to trees, soil, and water are keys to preventing
AIDS in Africa.

Michio and I are hopeful that the Congo will contribute to
the development of human health and a peaceful spirit and
spread all over the world. We hope that the Congo will dem-
onstrate the unification of modern contemporary medicine
and traditional natural medicine and daily macrobiotic eating
and living.

11: Erewhon Lost

"When we regard the clouds above,
Our souls are filled with fond desire,
To me the smoke of my dead love,
Seems rising from the funeral pyre."
—*The Tale of Genji*

IN HIS LECTURES in the United States and around the world, my husband spoke about biological degeneration. He said that the human race could die out from the spread of cancer, heart disease, arthritis, mental illness, and other sickness. He said that modern medicine's approach was superficial, addressing itself to symptoms rather than underlying causes. Everyone knew that nuclear war could wipe out the planet. There was nowhere to hide. But most people were not aware that humanity could destroy itself from within through improper diet. Michio compared macrobiotics to a modern-day Noah's Ark: "Only those who know how to control and manage their own health and destiny will survive the flood of unnatural, chemically processed foods." The best place to take refuge was Erewhon. A magical kingdom, based on whole grains and vegetables and principles of health, happiness, and peace, was spreading invisibly around the planet.

In the early 1970s, the medical and scientific associations continued to ignore or dismiss macrobiotics and the benefits of natural foods. They believed that the modern diet was the best ever developed. Calories, protein, and vitamins ruled. Except for rare diseases like scurvy, the American Medical Association held that there was no relation between food and health. They believed that disease resulted from poor sanitation, viral infection, or genetic mutation. Polio and smallpox had been wiped out. Surely a technological solution to cancer and other degenerative diseases was just around the corner. My husband's contention that macrobiotics could both prevent and relieve sicknesses that had eluded the best medical researchers was considered preposterous. Like the Cambridge police ten years earlier, many doctors and scientists saw him as a sorcerer or quack. Besides, everyone knew that health food was supposed to taste bad. Coupled with Zen fanaticism, society thought it was no wonder macrobiotic people were so thin and reserved. Our whole movement was regarded as a cult.

Natural foods had been widely available for nearly ten years. Thousands of people had improved their health. But they were mostly former hippies, peace marchers, back-to-the-landers, and college drop-outs. They had little influence on public opinion. Macrobiotics had not yet entered the mainstream of society. How were we to reach them? Through the East West Foundation we began public education and promotion. We held evening and weekend lectures in churches, schools, and community centers and invited the general public to attend. We also started seminars for doctors, nurses, and other medical professionals. We rented hotel space in downtown Boston, and my husband would lecture on Oriental medicine and philosophy.

The medical seminars were extremely popular. By now, relations with Peking had dramatically changed. After thirty years' hostility, America fell in love with China. After James Reston's emergency acupuncture treatment in Shanghai, everyone was fascinated with this ancient healing system. They wanted to know more about the Far Eastern view of life it was based on.

During our years in Boston, people increasingly came to see my husband for consultations. He was always careful to tell them that he was an educator, not a doctor. He offered them advice and guidance in their diet and way of life. But he left it entirely up to them whether to continue medical treatment. Whenever possible, he would cooperate with the family doctor or specialist if he or she was sympathetic to our approach. The sick friends who came to see us asked me to help prepare special dishes and menus. In my classes, I started to give workshops on medicinal cooking. I taught people how to prepare traditional home cares such as the ginger compress that had been used for thousands of years in the Far East.

During one of our East West Foundation planning meetings on macrobiotic education, I suggested that we target cancer. Among modern diseases, it was the most frightening. Every year the cancer societies reported victory was imminent. New drugs were being tested, and chemotherapy and radiation techniques had improved. Society was led to believe that it was only a matter of more time and money before a cure was found. But as the years went by, it became clear no such solution was in sight. The toll from cancer continued to mount. It now touched nearly every family in America. Like the Vietnam war, everyone knew deep inside that this was a war the nation would not win.

Many people started to attend our cancer-prevention seminars, including cancer patients and their families. Many of them had been declared terminally ill by the medical profession. In some cases, they had tried other alternatives such as juice fasts, raw foods, and large doses of vitamin C. By the time they came to us, many felt they had nothing to lose. They were depressed, confused, frightened. Often they came over the objection of their wife or husband or their children or doctor.

My husband embraced them all, regardless of their fears and doubts. He told them that "medically terminal" was often "macrobiotically hopeful." People whose condition was diagnosed late and were declared inoperable sometimes made more rapid progress with macrobiotics than those who had received medical treatment. However, Michio did not raise false hopes. Some cases, he noted, could not be relieved. The disease was too far progressed, the person lacked the will to live, or chemotherapy or other treatment had so weakened the body that recovery was unlikely. Nevertheless, even a short time eating macrobiotically was beneficial, he reassured them. The person's pain and discomfort eased. They felt more peaceful, and they usually died at home rather than in the hospital. The most important thing was proper cooking instruction, chewing well, keeping a bright, cheerful mind, and having the loving support of one's partner and family.

In addition to the medical profession, some macrobiotic friends opposed our cancer-prevention programs. They believed that macrobiotic cooking—humanity's highest art—should not be turned into a popular diet. They felt that macrobiotics was a highly refined way of life and could not be started apart from its cultural and philosophical foundation. Michio and I respected this view. The human potential movement was sweeping the country at this time, and we were wary of training programs that sought to transform people in a weekend or teach them values that took a lifetime to master. But we felt that macrobiotics was everyone's birthright. Macrobiotics was not Eastern or Western, but universal. It was not only for the spiritually developed, but for the foolish and the ignorant. Above all, it was for ordinary, suffering humanity.

By now, Michio was a great teacher. He saw clearly that his mission was to turn the entire world from self-destruction. But unlike most revolutionaries, he was infinitely patient. He would explain to a new friend over and over again how to cook miso or how to scrub each finger and toe with a towel soaked in hot ginger water. He would attend endless meetings at Erewhon, the restaurants, the East West Foundation, and *East West Journal*, discussing how to present macrobiotics in a clearer, less esoteric way. He helped devise creative solutions to their periodic money crises and helped resolve the personality conflicts that inevitably developed. Whatever people wanted Michio to do, he did in a spirit of service, thankfulness, and merry, good humor. He never put himself above anyone. No matter how difficult things became, he saw the endless balance of the Order of the Universe working itself out. He regarded everything as infinitely just and amusing.

Everyone came away marveling at how he had penetrated the heart of a matter or unified irreconcilable forces.

Many people with cancer who heard Michio were inspired to start macrobiotics and became better. We encouraged them to speak at our seminars and describe their experience to others. Their stories were written up in the *East West Journal* and the East West Foundation's *Case History Reports*. Told in simple, straightforward, everyday language by ordinary people, these accounts had a tremendous effect. For the first time, the average American family began to pay attention to macrobiotics. They heard the people next door—teachers, contractors, lawyers, housewives—speaking about the healing power of whole grains and vegetables. Still, the medical profession ignored our success. They said personal testimonials were "anecdotal" and worthless from a scientific point of view. Only carefully monitored case-control experiments would count. We offered to cooperate with the cancer societies but were told it wouldn't be ethical to start case-control studies unless there was evidence macrobiotics worked. It was a Catch-22.

The breakthrough came with Eugene Kohler. Jean was a middle-age professor of music at Ball State University in Richmond, Indiana. He had cancer of the pancreas. According to modern medicine, this type of cancer is incurable. There is no treatment other than pain-killers. Almost all pancreatic cancer patients die within six months to a year.

Jean Kohler was a very gentle, soft-spoken man. He was so modest that he waited a long time to come to Boston, not wanting to bother my husband with his problem. Gradually, thanks to the wonderful cooking and support of his wife, Mary Alice, Jean grew better and better on the macrobiotic diet. Eventually, he regained his vitality, and all signs of the tumor disappeared. In a spirit of gratitude, Jean decided to dedicate the rest of his life to spreading macrobiotics. He spoke to other cancer patients, wrote letters to newspapers and maga-zines, and gave interviews on radio and television. He gave benefit music concerts for macrobiotic centers, organized con-

ferences of cancer patients and their families, and labored
tirelessly to make this healing knowledge available to everyone who needed it.

Jean was an excellent speaker and influenced many friends.
His smiling eyes, calm, gentle manner, and obvious good
health disarmed the critics. From a scientific view, his was
a strong case. He had medical documentation. Besides, there
was no need of case-control studies for his type of cancer.
Almost no one had survived a tumor in the pancreas as long as
he did. But here he was, full of life, radiating joy and happiness. The medical establishment started to take notice.

Meanwhile, Frank Sacks, one of the young medical friends
who had attended my husband's lectures, started studying
the cholesterol levels and blood pressure values of macrobiotic people in Boston. At Harvard Medical School, Frank
and his colleagues found that macrobiotic people had the most
ideal blood quality of any group in modern society. The macrobiotic blood values were matched only by people in traditional societies where heart disease, cancer, and other degenerative diseases were unknown. The researchers were astonished. Several groups had better health than Americans as
a whole, including the Seventh Day Adventists and the
Mormons. But they had complex membership requirements
and belief systems, while the macrobiotic community had
none. Eating macrobiotic food was the only criterion, and
the average length on the diet was just over two years.
The researchers concluded that macrobiotics could serve as
an almost utopian model for modern society as a whole to
reverse heart disease, the nation's leading cause of death.

From a medical point of view, these were the case-control
studies macrobiotics needed to merit attention. Published in
the leading medical journals, including the *Journal of the
American Medical Association* and the *New England Journal
of Medicine*, they were taken seriously and had a big impact
on modern medicine. Dr. William Castelli came to our East
West Foundation conferences and endorsed our approach. He
was the director of the Framingham Heart Study, the nation's

oldest and most influential heart disease research project. He said macrobiotic people were in even better cardiovascular health than highly conditioned athletes in the famous Boston Marathon. Other leading doctors and medical friends also voiced their support. Macrobiotics was no longer a cult diet. It was modern civilization's best hope of health and survival.

In Washington, D.C., Michio and several friends from Erewhon, the East West Foundation, and *East West Journal* met with White House and congressional leaders. In 1977, the McGovern Report came out. Led by Senator George McGovern, the former Democratic presidential candidate, and Robert Dole, the Republican vice-presidential nominee, a blue-ribbon Senate panel linked heart disease, cancer, and other leading causes of death with the modern diet. In *Dietary Goals for the United States*, the Senators called for drastic reductions in consumption of animal food, sugar, and refined foods and substantial increases in whole grains, vegetables, and fresh fruits. The McGovern Report sent shock waves through the medical profession, the food industry, the public school system, and consumer interest groups. Despite some initial resistance from vested interests, the nation began to move in a more healthy direction. Within a few years, the wisdom of a low-fat, high-fiber diet became universally accepted. Senator McGovern subsequently endorsed Michio's major book, *The Cancer-Prevention Diet*, spelling out the macrobiotic approach to disease. The McGovern Report was the turning point in America's return to health and freedom. Though he had lost the presidency, George McGovern had earned an enduring place in history.

The Standard Macrobiotic Diet

During our time in Boston, our understanding continued to deepen and grow. My husband and I constantly refined our teaching and cooking methods. By the mid-1970s the macrobiotic way of eating in America was very different from that of earlier years.

In New York, we were beginners. The Ohsawas had not taught cooking at their school, and we had to learn for ourselves. In the beginning, I was very strict. Michio was always much more flexible. When we went out, I was content to order just a salad or pretend to eat what had been served. Michio enjoyed much more variety. He liked fish and seafood, as well as noodles. For the sake of being sociable, he would often eat what other people ate.

At home, I cooked Japanese style, using a lot of sea salt, miso, and tamari soy sauce. In Boston, as more young people studied with us, I started to cook more American and international style dishes. I also started to decrease the amount of seasoning I used. In his lectures and books, George Ohsawa had said that salt was the magician. A touch of salt, if used at the right time and in the right amount, controlled the smooth functioning of the kidneys and other organs. This was traditionally known. Improperly used, it could lead to physical and mental imbalance.

Like most Japanese macrobiotic friends. I had been using liberal amounts of salt. I made *gomashio* with 1 part salt to 4 parts sesame seeds. I used 1/4 teaspoon of salt for each cup of brown rice I prepared. I added almost 1 tablespoon of miso per cup of miso soup. In Japan, these are considered ordinary ratios. In America, however, they were much too high. This country is very dry compared to Japan. At meals, water is always brought to the table first here but never in Japan. Also, plenty of fresh salad is eaten here. While liquid and salad help to balance meat, the climate in the United States is generally more yang than in Japan. Much less salt and other seasonings are required to make daily balance.

Gradually, I began to reduce their use. Ultimately, I found that 1 part salt to 14 parts sesame seeds was more appropriate in this climate. I used only a pinch of sea salt per cup of rice and a teaspoon or less of miso per cup of soup. As our cooking changed more in harmony with the North American environment, our students grew steadier and more comfortable. Before, they had become yang very quickly and couldn't stay on the diet. After taking too much salt, tamari soy sauce, or miso, they would binge. They would be very strict and then go out and eat ice cream, chocolate cake, and candy. Mentally and psychologically, there were also many ups and downs. When you become too yang, you become very rigid, stubborn, and intolerant of others. You become so wound up that you change jobs, partners, and places to live frequently. You get tighter and tighter until you explode and swing over to the other extreme—too much yin.

In addition to seasonings, we found that other dietary modifications were necessary. In Japan, we usually don't have desserts. Instead of sweets, we serve pickles at tea time. In New York, I made a few Japanese sweet dishes for dessert using azuki beans and chestnuts. In Boston, I found that many American friends were not satisfied without dessert. And they weren't satisfied with Japanese style sweet dishes. In Cambridge, I found that my students were expert at making delicious natural desserts without sugar, white flour, and other unsuitable ingredients. In one of my first classes, I turned the kitchen over to one of the Ruhani Satsang ladies. She showed us all how to make delicious whole wheat pie crust. I used her recipes for a long time.

From my side, it sometimes seems that macrobiotic food is becoming too yin! Americans are very talented at turning yang into yin, like inventing tofu cheesecake. In Japan, we never imagined making tofu sweet or using it to make cakes and desserts. Eaten cold, raw, or mixed with sweeteners, tofu can lead to lower sexual vitality.

Later when we lived on Gardner Road in Brookline, I used to make sourdough bread. Americans and Europeans can take more bread and hard baked flour products than Japanese. The same thing with fruit. In the beginning, we minimized fruit. George Ohsawa taught that fruits were too yin for ordinary use. Norio, my oldest son, recalls tasting an apple for the first time at school when he was six years old.

Over the years, many such changes occurred. The kinds of vegetables we ate broadened. Cooking styles lightened up.

Before we used a lot of oil to balance all the salt we took in. We were always making tempura, deep-fried foods, and croquettes. In Boston, we started experimenting with good quality, traditional foods from around the world. I incorporated corn dishes from Latin America, cracked grains from the Middle East, and tempeh from Indonesia into my menus. The Seventh Inn, Sanae, and Open Sesame widened their selection and lightened their cooking styles. The public responded. Macrobiotic food was now varied and delicious as well as good for you. From Boston, this trend rippled across the country.

In his lectures and books, Michio began introducing the Standard Macrobiotic Diet. This was not a single diet but a flexible dietary approach that everyone could use to find the diet best suited for themselves. It involved applying common principles of food selection and preparation to different environments, climates, levels of activity, conditions of health, and everchanging personal needs. The standard by which he measured our basic human quality was 1) physical health, 2) a calm, peaceful mind, and 3) spiritual development. A way of eating that produced these qualities was ideal. In a four-season climate such as most of the United States, the Standard Diet by daily volume of food consumed included 50 to 60 percent whole cereal grains; 5 to 10 percent soup, including miso soup and others; 25 to 30 percent vegetables, consisting of many varieties and cooked in many ways; and 10 to 15 percent beans, bean products, and seaweed. For those in usual good health, fish or seafood could be enjoyed two or three times a week; fruit and sometimes juice or cider could be eaten occasionally; seeds and nuts could be prepared as snacks; and desserts could be prepared several times a week sweetened with fruit or good quality natural sweetener such as rice syrup or barley malt. A wide range of condiments, garnishes, pickles, and beverages could also be eaten daily.

For people with cancer or other sicknesses, my husband recommended a more limited form of the diet. For several months up to a year or two or longer, they may need to avoid or restrict fish, fruit, nuts, desserts, and many of the other supplemental foods. For people who had eaten a lot of meat, chicken, and other yang foods, it was especially important to limit salt and seasoning. For those who had taken too much sugar, sweets, soft drinks, and other yin items, it was necessary to reduce oil. Many sick friends came to my cooking classes. This naturally helped me understand better the proper use of these subtle ingredients.

As presented by Michio, the Standard Diet offered almost infinite variety and enjoyment. He said that the main reason people leave macrobiotics is a lack of variety in their cooking. Day after day, people eat the same thing prepared in the same way and get tired of the food. He was fond of telling people that there were at least a thousand ways to cook brown rice. By varying the kind of rice (short, middle, long grain, sweet), the type of seasoning (salt, tamari, *umeboshi*, miso), the method of cooking (pressure-cooking, boiling, roasting), and from time to time adding a small portion of other grains or beans (corn, barley, wild rice, azuki beans, chestnuts, lotus seeds), an endless variety of dishes could be made.

Over time, the Standard Diet began to displace the older, Japanese-style of macrobiotic cooking. Macrobiotic cookbooks no longer copied Ohsawa's salty style of cooking or observed the ten levels of eating in *Zen Macrobiotics*. The famous number 7 all-brown rice diet became a special fasting diet, not an everyday diet. It was used for only brief periods for healing purposes or for spiritual development. The scientific and medical profession found the new style of macrobiotics much more balanced. Professor Frederick Stare, our toughest critic, changed his attitude. In an article favorable to macrobiotics in *The New York Times*, the chairman of the nutrition department at Harvard was quoted as saying the macrobiotic diet, as currently taught, was completely nutritious.

Parents, teachers, and school lunch program administrators all welcomed the changes. As macrobiotic people ate more widely, their view of life and way of relating to other people also improved. People became more open and understanding of others. Macrobiotics also began to outgrow its Japanese

242

cultural parentage. Many terms for foods from Japan that had no English equivalent, such as "tamari," "miso," and "tofu," entered the American vocabulary. But common foods available here, such as carrots, burdock, and barley, were no longer referred to by their Japanese names. When my husband wrote his big book on cancer, an amusing situation arose. A large publisher in Tokyo wanted to translate it into Japanese but complained the recipes and menus were too American. The editors asked him to substitute foods that were more familiar to Japanese people. Macrobiotics had truly become a marriage of East and West!

Troubles at Erewhon

As modern society moved closer to macrobiotics, macrobiotics moved closer to modern society. This was especially true at Erewhon. What began as a small family business grew into a giant corporation. From South Boston, Erewhon moved to new headquarters in Cambridge. The workforce doubled, warehouse space quadrupled, and earnings soared.

In the beginning, the staff consisted of our students. They were young, inexperienced, and unskilled. But they had poetry and passion. Stimulated by Michio's lectures and our dreams, they hoped to change the world. They lived in study houses and walked or rode bicycles to work. If there was no money, no matter. They worked for nothing. On weekends they might make some spending money by taking a stack of *East West Journals* to sell on the Boston Common or Harvard Square. They reminded me of sprouting grasses. In watching them, I saw myself twenty-five years earlier in Tokyo selling the World Government newspaper on Tokyo subway platforms.

As Erewhon grew, the revenue that came in from sales was all put back into expansion. As chairman and owner respectively, my husband and I had overall control of the company. In practice, we left day-to-day administration to a president and managers so that we could be free to concentrate on our teaching and travels. Still, we played a direct role in maintaining high quality standards for products, selecting new items to import, and developing new goods to manufacture.

In order to remain competitive with other natural foods distributors, Erewhon started to sell things such as cheese, ice cream, bananas and pineapples, and vitamins. There was continuing debate within the company and within the macrobiotic community about the wisdom of such a policy. Some people felt that these foods were harmful to health per se and should not be encouraged. Others felt that natural foods shoppers needed to be educated gradually. According to this view, it was unrealistic to expect everyone to become macrobiotic overnight. So long as people were eating dairy food, tropical vegetables, vitamin supplements, and other modern foods, they should have the option of the best quality available. Besides, many of these items, especially the vitamins and beauty products, had the highest profits. Money made from these products could be put into developing new macrobiotic products.

Similar debates went on at the restaurants and at *East West Journal* about how flexible to be in matters of cooking or editorial content, in advertising, and in general presentation of macrobiotics to the public. When asked for our advice, my husband and I always suggested a middle course. We felt it was essential to maintain a macrobiotic focus to our enterprises. But we felt it was impractical to expect other people to change all at once. The different way of viewing things was just another example of yin and yang. More yin friends were concerned with quality, content, and aesthetic appeal. More yang friends stressed quantity, form, and practical results. We were happy to see Erewhon and the *East West Journal* serve as the vanguard of the larger natural foods movement, new age community, and holistic health profession. There was room for both principle and profit. The important thing was for principle to lead, not the other way around.

As Erewhon expanded, new jobs opened up in the warehouse and retail stores. There were not enough macrobiotic people to fill all the positions. Many people were hired who had a loose interest in natural foods but no real commitment to studying with us. By the mid-seventies, internal conflict had erupted throughout the company. The workers, many of whom were nonmacrobiotic, felt they were paid poorly and passed over for promotion. The managers, most of whom were macrobiotic, felt they had earned their higher salaries and status because of their commitment to our educational activities. The managers felt some of the workers were unreliable, inefficient, or imbalanced. They made dietary recommendations and suggested the nonmacrobiotic people attend lectures and seminars. This only increased polarity.

My husband and I were largely unaware of these developments. When we came back from Europe one time, we learned of an effort to create a union in Erewhon. I couldn't believe it. In Japan, there had been a teachers' union after the war. My classmates who were now teachers themselves all agreed that it had contributed to the decline in the quality of teaching. In the old days, such revolts had also occurred. I was reminded of the peasant uprisings against the lord of the clan in medieval Japan. In America, of course, strikes were a regular occurrence. But the thought of a union in Erewhon had never occurred to us. We were deeply shocked.

The essense of our teachings is gratitude for nature and respect for other people. "From one grain, ten thousand grains." If macrobiotics has a motto, it is this saying. Endlessly give back what the universe has given to you. From the endless multiplication of seeds in the fields to the infinite expansion of galaxies, this is the Order of the Universe. From this perspective, the union was concerned with taking, not giving. Even some of our students joined. Abuses certainly existed. Some of the managers were too yang—arrogant and insensitive. We hoped differences could be worked out peacefully. Discussions, negotiations, and community meetings followed. But the split went too deep. The union was formed. It later joined the Teamsters. We were saddened.

Erewhon began to get in trouble from another quarter. To

handle the huge volume of orders, Erewhon had to constantly expand its machinery, lease new trucks, install new communications equipment, and take out more bank loans. Pretty soon the business was so complicated that we had to hire accountants and marketing executives to run things. These people were not macrobiotic, but they had experience in the world of business. They were adept at sales, knew how to keep inventory, and balance the books. They knew how to negotiate with banks. In return for high salaries, they promised order, efficiency, and smoother operations. We started to relax.

By 1980, however, Erewhon's financial situation had worsened. The company had become overextended. It had expanded so rapidly that it could no longer pay its bills on time. Much of its money was being used to pay the interest on large bank loans taken to finance its expansion. High inflation and high interest rates of the time contributed to this deficit. Wholesalers, farmers, manufacturers, importers, and other trade partners began to reduce their credit. Erewhon's debts mounted. New loans were taken out at higher interest rates.

By the following summer, the situation became precarious. My husband and I were in Innsbruck, Austria, teaching when we heard the news. For the rest of our seminars there, Michio was busy contacting investors and brokers to help prevent collapse. Days and evenings he would lecture, nights he would be on the telephone till daybreak. I don't think he hardly slept for almost two weeks. For us, it was not a matter of saving our personal business. It was saving the leader of the whole natural foods movement. The future of humanity depended on the continuing availability of good food. If we sold Erewhon, as some people suggested, we could no longer guarantee the basic quality of the foods it distributed.

The immediate crisis came about when Erewhon's accountant had to go to jail. He was a professional and had not studied with us. We trusted the judgment of Erewhon's president at the time and agreed to hire him. Unknown to us, he had been involved in some previous criminal case and was sent to Lewisberg Penitentiary in Pennsylvania. Our intuition should have been sharper. In any event, Erewhon didn't have anyone to replace him. When we returned to Boston, Michio took over everything. He went to Erewhon every day to manage things. He found many mistakes and set about making improvements, but by then it was too late.

In the fall, the company could no longer meet its payroll. Production and distribution came to a halt. The lawyers intervened. Nearly every day we met with Morris Kirsner, our lawyer, and attorneys for creditors. We met downtown on State Street in plush offices on the top floor of a skyscraper. On November 20, we filed for temporary bankruptcy under Chapter 11 of the laws of Massachusetts.

At that time I was sole owner of Erewhon. When I finally signed the paper for Chapter 11, strong tears unexpectedly came down from my eyes. I couldn't stop weeping. Past memories flooded my mind. I apologized to all the creditors who lost money, especially Mr. Kazama of Mitoku, and the farmers who had faith in us and many of our young friends who had devoted themselves to the cause of healthy food. One by one their faces appeared before my mind's eye like a thunderbolt. When I stopped crying, I noticed that all the lawyers had left the room. My husband alone remained.

Under Chapter 11, Erewhon's management was put under the authority of a special court-appointed officer. We had three months to reorganize the company. The meetings with the lawyers continued.

Winter was just beginning. I used to drive downtown via Storrow Drive or Memorial Parkway. Sometimes I would pick up my husband at the Erewhon warehouse in Cambridge near the Science Museum. On the way, I noticed the leaves on the willow trees along the Charles River. Leaves from the other trees had already fallen. But the willow was still holding on, its leaves still golden.

Winter passed and spring came. The lawyers' meetings continued. Progress was slow. Driving along the river, I noticed that the willow leaves were the first to come forth. I observed many people jogging up and down the Esplanade. I recalled my days at college organizing the gymnastics club. How I envied the runners' freedom.

Finally, a deal was struck. Nature Food Centers, a chain of health food stores, would take over Erewhon. In exchange for assuming its debts, it would invest money in the company, maintain quality standards, and retain Michio as an adviser to the board.

I really appreciated many people's support, but we had to go that way. Tremendous orders were still coming in, and only 40 percent could be filled. We felt it was better to turn the company over to someone who could keep it going than to go out of business entirely.

In the days and weeks after, I thanked everyone who had helped us, financially and otherwise. I apologized to all the people who were hurt when Erewhon couldn't pay its bills. The loss of Erewhon was the most difficult period of our life.

From a business standpoint, we had failed, but from an educational view it was a great success. Thanks to Erewhon, everyone in this country and in many parts of the world knows the concept of natural foods. The people who worked and studied there went on to found other macrobiotic and whole foods companies, ensuring continued availability of good food. Other friends who worked there are now contributing to society in many other ways and will be the leaders of the future world. Like a seed that dies in the ground and gives birth to new life, Erewhon had accomplished its purpose.

To our pleasant surprise, the company itself continued to prosper. Though it was not run by macrobiotic friends, the new owners were health-conscious and generally maintained high standards. Five years later, they sold it to someone else, and now it is reportedly moving its main warehouse to Omaha, Nebraska.

Originally Erewhon was like a young sprouting grass or flower of spring. That happy Erewhon exists now only in our memories. But the dream of making available beautiful, natural food to everyone at a fair price will continue endlessly. Without the best quality food, we can never achieve our true dream of one peaceful world.

12: The Spirit of Family Harmony

"All within the four seas are brothers." —Confucius

THE RELATION between man and woman is eternally fascinating. In traditional societies, woman takes care of the home, while man provides the income. In Japan, which still follows the traditional role of the sexes, it looks like man dominates and woman is following. But many times, woman is actually the boss. She controls the children, the family, and the purse strings. The Japanese husband puts his complete trust in his wife's hands and customarily gives his whole salary to her. She then handles all household expenses and gives him a small allowance for his daily needs. Of course, in some cases the husband controls the family finances day-to-day, too. From the outside, it appears that woman is the servant of man in the East. From the inside, it is the other way around.

According to traditional understanding, this way of managing relations developed because of basic physiological differences between man and woman. Governed more by inward coming, yang centripetal force from the heavens, man is more suited to physical and social activity. He is bigger, stronger, and requires slightly stronger cooking, more volume of food, and, if desired, occasional animal food in his diet. Woman, on the other hand, is governed more by outward moving, yin centrifugal force from the rotation of the earth. She is more suited to aesthetic and mental activity. She is smaller, more delicate, and requires slightly lighter cooking, less volume of food, and little or no animal food in her diet. The slight difference between the sexes is the source of their attraction. When woman eats too much animal food, or when man eats too many salads or sweets, the magnet is dulled.

Many young people today lose their sensitivity by attending coeducational colleges. Both my husband and I attended college with only the same sex. The experience contributed to our attraction. Too much explicitness also destroys happiness between the sexes. The sexual revolution has taken the mystery out of sex and love.

Biologically, woman is more developed than man and can give birth and nourish her child. In traditional families, she has assumed charge of preparing the food for the whole family. Cooking is the highest art, since it creates and shapes daily life. The person in charge of the kitchen has the responsibility for the whole family's health and happiness. In ages past, it was recognized that woman had the higher intellectual, aesthetic, and spiritual capacity.

In our case, my husband and I did not really follow the Japanese style. Sometimes I take the initiative in cultural and business activity and he follows my lead. However, my outside efforts are just an extension of my home. All of our enterprises have been run on a family basis. Meetings with staff, teachers, managers, suppliers, accountants, publishers, boards of directors, and attorneys have been informal. Often we meet in the living room of our home in Brookline. We always serve delicious, healthful macrobiotic food such as sushi, *ohagi*, noodles, or tempura. Still, disagreements occur from time to time about the best way to proceed. But everyone feels united in sharing a common dream, and we are able to proceed harmoniously.

Many times after we came to Boston the topic of women's liberation came up. From the outside, it appeared that macrobiotics was following the Oriental style: the ladies were in the kitchen, the men were out dealing with society. In the early years especially, I was busy with the children, and it looked like I was in the home and not going out. Many of our students followed this model, not realizing that my husband and

I did much of our business at home and together discussed all
important decisions.

From the beginning of women's liberation, I could never
understand why they made this an issue. Macrobiotic ladies
held many discussions on the subject. I always told them,
"We are already leading men. If we don't like the way they
are treating us, we can change them. Through our day-to-day
cooking, we can change their minds and behavior. The key is
in our hands. Whether they are angels or devils is entirely
up to us."

Of course, because of eating the modern diet for many
years, men and women have both become imbalanced. Practically speaking, even among macrobiotic friends, it sometimes
takes a long time to let go of past ways of thinking and acting.
Also, it takes experience to be able to cook intuitively and
really change your family. For many young macrobiotic ladies,
it is simply a question of time and practice. Once their own
health and judgment are restored, it is very easy to influence
others.

The center of human life is the lady's *hara*. The hara is the
vital energy center of the body. It is located deep in the intestines. There, in the womb, pregnancy takes place. There creation starts and life begins. To give birth to a baby requires
strength. For millions of years, this process hasn't changed.
A woman today who carries a baby becomes very strong. Man
cannot compete with her. In fact, man today no longer rides
horseback, farms, or catches the family's daily food. He often
drives to work, uses a computer at the office, and comes home
and watches TV. There are less and less physical challenges
and outlets for him. This is a big problem. Modern man is
becoming too weak. Woman likes a man who has energy for
the day like a hungry tiger.

Modern man should balance his life with some rigorous
activity. In addition to sports or outdoor activities, he can
help woman in the house, cleaning, vacuuming, and taking
care of the children. A home with children is busier than
an office. Man too should learn to cook and occasionally cook

for his family to give woman a rest. He should frequently take her out.

Modern woman has a big responsibility. But she needs to awaken and discover herself within the larger Order of the Universe. Everything changes. That is the key. Pregnancy really creates new offspring. Whether intended or not, woman should still put her whole effort into preparing for her new child. Breastfeeding is also essential. It not only secures her baby's future health, it also creates love between them. From nursing my children I really began to understand the order of nature and the meaning of care and nourishment. By bringing up her children in a natural way, woman can change society. The shortest way to true world peace leads through the kitchen. Wars can be stopped by raising children with strong, healthy bodies and calm, peaceful minds.

There are many ways for man to serve society and bring happiness to his family. He can participate in natural or organic agriculture, natural foods manufacturing or distribution, and managing natural foods stores, co-ops, or restaurants. He can also become a teacher, counselor, writer, artist, or architect. There are many ways to create natural order and make a better world. Everyone will be happy and satisfied. If the total view is clear, anything is all right. Sometimes man may want to be at home and take care of the family, and woman may go out and work. Once both people are eating well, they can be flexible. The whole purpose of macrobiotics is to be free. If they truly understand yin and yang, man and woman can do whatever they want, automatically, spontaneously, and without complaint. In my home, I generally take the lead, while my husband follows. He is more interested in teaching and counseling and prefers to leave practical matters to others.

America is the leader of the modern world. It is a large and diverse land. The rest of the world looks to us for leadership in man/woman relations as well as food, technology, and entertainment. The number one priority is producing good quality food in this country instead of depending on imports

from Japan and other countries. There are many things we
can do for ourselves and society. If man and woman combine
their efforts, the whole world can be turned from cancer,
AIDS, poverty, and war. Our influence as mothers and as
macrobiotic women can be very great.

My Children

I conceived my first child on a visit to England. When we
returned to the United States we had no money, and my husband had no job. It was a very difficult time. We were able
to buy River Rice, Quaker Oats, and Wolff's Buckwheat at
the supermarket. We were also able to get seaweed and buckwheat noodles from a Japanese store. During my first pregnancy I couldn't stop eating fruit in the summer. Two nonmacrobiotic ladies from Hawaii were staying in our apartment
at the time. They kept grapefruit in the refrigerator, and one
day, before I realized it, I had eaten one of them. It was as
if someone else had put it in my mouth. Lilly, my first child,
was born in the women's hospital near Columbia University.
I always carried her with me when I went out, even to the
movies.

I conceived again after nine months. My sister told me that
while I was breastfeeding I could not get pregnant. But I had
several periods before then. A friend asked me if I had used
any protection, and in surprise, I said no. She told me how to
use a diaphragm which I used a couple of times and then gave
up. It was too complicated.

When I was carrying my second child I craved buckwheat.
In Japan we usually eat buckwheat in noodles rather than
taking it as a grain. As a child, soba always gave me a headache and I never enjoyed it. But I started to like buckwheat
groats very much, especially when I fried them with vegetables like onions and celery and added a little chopped raw
vegetable as a garnish. They had a rich, delicious taste, and
the colorful array of carrots, radishes, burdock, and parsley
reminded me of a beautiful Japanese silkscreen print.

I ate buckwheat practically every day for a time, and as a result, Norio, my second child was very yang, very active —like a Russian Cossack. Although he is pretty smart, he never liked to study, and he dropped out of high school. George Ohsawa said that if you want your children to study, better not give them buckwheat, but if you want them to be active buckwheat is very good.

Norio's birth was quick and without trouble. After I came back from the hospital, Lilly was very surprised. Until that time, she had always been with me and was still sleeping in my bed. When she saw the new baby getting milk, she was shocked and saddened. She tried to push the baby away. But soon she accepted it, and they grew up as good playmates.

In New York, Norio and Lilly grew up in relatively good health. Once a painter left some paint in the children's room. That night Norio had an allergic reaction to the paint. His whole body broke out in red, and his skin became rough. He could hardly breathe, and we wondered if he would survive. Lilly was not affected by the paint at all. I continued breast-feeding Norio, and fortunately he got well. In a week, his hard skin dried up, and he could breathe normally again. But it gave us quiet a scare. Our big, fat baby had become very skinny. It was a shocking introduction to the effects of toxic chemicals used in the modern house.

At the hospital, I was given a course in how to immerse my new babies in warm water very quickly. In Japan we actually dip the baby in the water after birth. We hold the head near the ears, and the body floats easily. For at least a week after the birth, a midwife comes herself to wash the baby, usually in the morning. After that, the grandmother, sister, or someone else takes care of washing the baby. After the bath, the baby sleeps peacefully, and each day a little more water is needed as the baby starts to grow. Also, during delivery, when the mother begins to experience contractions, it is important to prepare hot water for the birth. In our case, my husband liked to wash the babies when they were young. Sometimes three or four children were together with him in the bathtub, or other times I would bring the babies one by one while he was in the tub. In this way he was a very big help.

When I became pregnant again, it was a very busy time. In addition to caring for my first two children, we had a store in Greenwich Village, and I had to go there to help out. My third child, Haruo, was born very simply. In structure, his head was bigger than the other children's. We worried about his proportions, but he grew up nicely without any trouble. He followed his brother and sister, playing quietly.

Norio was very active but shy. He hid behind my skirt when guests came. When I took him to kindergarten, I had to stay with him for an hour until he started playing with the other children. One day after school, a mother of one of his classmates told me that the day before her son reported that Norio had spoken in class. She asked her son what he had said. He said Norio had just laughed. He spoke so rarely it was the big news of the day. After we got a television, both Lilly's and Norio's English improved. Until then we had been speaking Japanese at home.

The next year Lilly and Norio attended the same class. The teacher reported that sometimes he talked too much. We thought being in the same room with his sister caused him to speak up more. Haruo, meanwhile, entered kindergarten. He had grown up watching TV, so English was never a problem. He was always a model student. One time, his teacher told me, "I'm very happy today." I asked her why. She said, "Haruo made a mistake in class. He is never wrong. I am relieved. This shows he's normal."

When the children were small, we encouraged them to study music. At age five, Lilly began to practice piano at a nearby music school. I wanted Norio to study violin. He was not very interested, though he took some piano lessons too. Lilly has studied music since that time.

When the children were older, I started teaching macrobiotic cooking. In some of my classes, I experimented with making whole wheat bread. It was before we knew about sourdough, so I used yeast. The children enjoyed the bread very much. One day, while driving from school, we passed a movie theater. Norio read the name of the movie playing in a loud voice. I asked Lilly to read the marquee too, but she couldn't see the letters. I was shocked. Back home, we discovered she had a problem with her eyesight. My husband and I tried to find out the cause of her problems. We finally figured out that it was from the yeast in the bread and also possibly from too much salt and overeating. These foods were affecting her liver, which in turn governed the eyes according to traditional Oriental medicine. Although she got glasses, her eyesight improved when we cut out yeasted bread and reduced her salt.

When they were young, I made lunch for my children to take to school. I made mostly rice balls. They enjoyed them, but in the third grade they became aware that they were eating differently from their classmates. They hesitated to take their lunch any more. I told them, "I don't want you to eat the school lunch. If you don't take a lunch from home, you will be very hungry." They said it would be all right. They would go to the library and read for 15 or 20 minutes instead of eating lunch. After school, they would have a mid-afternoon meal at home.

I think my children started to binge at this time, eating cheese and some other foods we didn't normally use at home. Norio recalls eating candy for the first time while we were living in Queens. One day I took him to the barbershop for a haircut. Afterward, the barber offered him a lollipop. I told the barber that I didn't want my son to eat sugar. The next time he needed a haircut, Norio went by himself and came home with four or five lollipops. He ate them in secret and loved them. Later he acquired some Life-Savers and brought them back to his brother and sister. Looking back, he said he felt like the serpent in the Garden of Eden offering forbidden fruit. He said they all found the candy delicious. When I discovered the candy, I took it away but didn't scold them. I told my children it wasn't good for their health and it was better not to eat.

Another time, Lilly was in junior high in Wellesley. She came back, and I noticed that the tip of her nose was purple and swollen. I asked her what had happened. She hadn't noticed and felt no pain. She went to look in mirror and was so surprised.

"Did anything special happen?" I quizzed her.

She then recalled that some friends insisted that she eat some ice cream with them. She had never eaten ice cream before.

"I put just a spoonful in my mouth. I didn't like it and spit it out," she explained.

It wasn't until my children were older that I realized how hard it was for them to grow up macrobiotic. Haruo later wrote the foreword to a book on macrobiotic childcare and described how embarrassed he felt eating differently from his friends. I was really surprised when I read his article. I found macrobiotic children in general had similar views. Now I think it's important for parents to make lunches for their children that look like what their friends are eating. In my classes, I now recommend tempeh burgers, seitan sandwiches, and other good quality items that can be made for children and which they very much enjoy to take and share with their friends.

Lilly was not sociable but made many friends among the macrobiotic people who came to study and live with us. She learned to cook very well and has helped me with the recipes for several medicinal cookbooks. In Boston, she went to a couple of music schools, including Berkelee School of Music, and became a talented pianist and composer. She went on to study further in Los Angeles. She also enjoys photography and kept our family's picture albums. She married once to a nice young man who had studied with us, but unfortunately it didn't last. I hope she will marry again.

Norio continued to be very active. As a child, he was interested in vehicles of all kinds and liked to travel. He loved trolley cars, ferryboats, and bicycles. At school, when asked to draw something, he would always draw a beautiful boat or car. One time he made a scale-model replica of a Boston trolley car. It had the same number of seats, and even the ads inside were exactly the same. It was marvelous. Norio also liked to ride his bicycle. He thought nothing of riding 150 miles from Boston to our summer program in Amherst and back. Once he rode his bike across the country. For several years, he worked as dispatcher for the taxi company in Brookline. Recently, he has driven trucks and buses. He drove a school bus in Connecticut and a big commercial bus for the Peter Pan lines. He also enjoys cars and for a while had a Saab he prized.

For Norio, relationships, like jobs, have often changed. He was born in a water year and because of his strong, floating constitution and character, he always seems to be looking for a new partner. Norio married a beautiful American lady named Candace who came to Boston to study macrobiotics. They divorced after seven years. I miss her very much. I don't know why they separated, but they didn't have a baby or I think they would still be together. After the divorce, he remarried, had a beautiful daughter, Liana, but unfortunately the marriage didn't last. Now he is taking care of his daughter and doing very well.

Norio helped managed Ghinga, the restaurant we established in Stockbridge. His dream is to establish a transportation business. He is now studying at the Kushi Institute., starting from the beginning. I hope he will provide transportation for macrobiotics and the whole world and make better communication between small countries and villages.

Compared to Norio and the other children, Haruo was physically the most delicate. We were always very careful of his physical condition and watched over him. As a child, he loved sports. He was crazy about baseball and collected almost five thousand baseball cards. He very much liked to attend Red Sox games in Boston. His father and I never went to sporting events. Occasionally we would play ball or jump rope with the children, and it reminded me when I was a star pitcher on our softball team in college.

While growing up, I never saw my children fighting. Once or twice, they would tussle, but they never really got angry or upset with each other. Shortly after we moved to Brookline, I started cooking with maple syrup for the first time. I noticed that after I gave it to Haruo, he started arguing with his brothers. He was ordinarily very quiet and well behaved. I was shocked at the strong reaction the maple syrup produced. I scolded him and told him not to be so aggressive. After dinner, he left the house. It was the first time he had ever been scolded. I knew he was upset. I followed him, ducking behind trees and bushes. I was worried and thought he might run away. But he went up the hill, made a big circle, and came back home. I was so relieved. Since then I have used maple syrup very, very sparingly.

The East West Foundation started seminars at Amherst College every summer. Located near the Berkshire mountains of western Massachusetts, the campus was very beautiful, and everyone thoroughly enjoyed it. From childhood, I had known about Amherst. A famous educator from Amherst, Dr. Clarke, went to Japan and taught at Hokkaido University. His motto, "Boys, be ambitious," is known throughout Japan. When Haruo was ready to apply to college, his father and I were very pleased when he decided to go to Amherst.

Before he arrived to begin his studies, I called the college officials. I told them, "My son cannot eat regular cafeteria food." I said I'd like to rent a house and cook for him or send a cook because he had never eaten away from home before. They said, "Please wait two weeks, because we are going to open a vegetarian, natural foods dining room for students who want to eat in this way." We were surprised and delighted that the school had listened to our request. Almost from the very beginning, there were about 150 students eating there! I arranged to supply the cafeteria natural foods from Erewhon. I sent our head cook from Sanae to Amherst, and he showed them how to prepare brown rice, miso soup, and other dishes. The natural foods movement was just about ten years old. Other colleges around the country began serving brown rice in their cafeterias. The benefits were already coming back to my son. I felt we had made a real revolution. From my experience, I can strongly recommend that parents concerned about their children's health join together and talk with the school officials about changing their cafeteria menus.

At college, Haruo applied to become an exchange student at Dōshisha University, Amherst's sister college in Kyoto, Japan. In preparing for his journey, he became very active and got too yang. I asked him to delay the trip, but he already had bought his ticket. In Japan he got jaundice. Some Japanese macrobiotic friends took care of him. They made dietary adjustments, giving him apple juice and shiitake mushrooms. The acute liver trouble cleared up. He stayed with Mr. and Mrs. Yoshida, a macrobiotic family in Kyoto who ran a kindergarten, and had a wonderful time.

From Amherst, Haruo went on to graduate study at the Harvard School of Public Health. He had always been very conscientious about his diet and wanted to integrate macrobiotic teachings with modern nutritional findings. He got a doctorate and became friends with Dr. Stare, chairman of the Harvard Department of Nutrition and his father's biggest critic. At Harvard, Haruo became involved in research on diet and heart disease and one year was invited to speak at the American Heart Association's annual convention in California. The excellence of his research was also recognized by *The New England Journal of Medicine*, which published a study on diet and heart disease he wrote. For several years he worked in the epidemiology department of the University of Minnesota School of Public Health. While in graduate school, Haruo married a beautiful young woman named Gabriele, who came to the Kushi Institute from Germany. They have a lovely daughter, Angelica. Haruo has taken the lead in unifying modern science and medicine with macrobiotics. He has even asked his father to stop coffee and cigarettes! Haruo and Gabriele have also been very active in peace education with Physicians for Social Responsibility and other social action groups, and he became chairperson of the Peace Caucus of the American Public Health Association.

Yoshio, my third son, was born in New York shortly before we moved to New England. Nicknamed Phiya, he was also on the quiet side like Haruo, but sometimes he showed strong wishes and was very curious and inventive. One day in Cambridge, while he was still a baby, we heard him crying in his room. My husband and I dashed upstairs and found a portion of his intestine protruding through the abdomen. We thought maybe he had injured himself on a pin or nail. Instinctively, I ran to the kitchen and grated some fresh gingerroot. I put about a half teaspoon of ginger in a cup of bancha tea and added one or two drops of tamari soy sauce. I ran upstairs and while Michio held him put some liquid to his mouth. As soon as the tea touched his lips, the intestinal tissue started to withdraw. In less than a second it disappeared. He had not taken one spoonful of the tea, just a drop. Michio and I were amazed. We knew that ginger was a traditional home remedy in the Far East, but that was the first time we had seen just how powerful it was. Phiya was all right after that.

When we first came to Boston, I would sometimes visit the Matson Academy of Karate where our first lecture was held. Bob Felt, one of our students, was teaching karate. I joined with all my children to practice. Phiya was the youngest, but he put his whole self into following the others. It was fun to watch.

Growing up, Phiya and Hisao, his younger brother, always went with us to attend summer camp in Europe. One time, Phiya met a lovely French girl there named Veronique. Her father was a yoga teacher and helped organize our first macrobiotic seminar in France. After high school, Phiya planned to go to Hampshire College but decided to take a year off. He went to Paris instead where Veronique was living. They married. He was only nineteen, she was twenty. They came back to Boston. We encouraged them to go back to college, but a baby came, and they were unable to finish school. Phiya went on to work at Open Sesame Restaurant and the East West Foundation, where he became the director, organizing seminars and summer camps. We were very happy with his devotion to macrobiotic activities and the three lovely sons he and Veronique raised. Recently, Phiya and his wife have had some difficulties and separated. I feel very sad for my grandchildren. When children are small, their problems remain small. When they grow, their problems also grow bigger. Life is an endless study of how to adapt to changing conditions, trying not to push one's own ideas but accepting life's difficulties and changes with gratitude.

Hisao, my last child, has always been very happy. When he was three years old, he fell down and hurt his knee. I took him to Los Angeles for a special massage treatment. Bill Tara would drive us from Los Angeles to San Francisco along the Pacific coastline. While driving past Big Sur, Hisao kept saying, "Tomorrow never comes. Right, Mommy?" He kept repeating this question over and over. I still remember his beautiful words. At home his father and I would often be busy and use expressions such as "OK, I will give it to you tomorrow," or "Wait until tomorrow." But Hisao saw clearly that tomorrow would never come.

Growing up, Hisao seemed most comfortable of all the children with our way of life. He is also the most social of the children. He liked to invite friends home and make noodles for them, or he would give them mochi and tell them it was some type of cheese. In high school he was captain of his track team. In his senior year, he had a party at our house in Brookline and invited his friends to come. About two hundred teenagers turned up. I was wary beforehand, but everything went smoothly. I danced with them and was pleased they did not drink. They were happy and quiet.

Hisao is now in college and took time off to visit his relatives in Japan and study the culture of the East. He has also been to Europe. It is too soon to know what direction he will go in. But George Ohsawa used to say that while the oldest child was often physically the strongest, the youngest one tended to be the most mentally active. I hope Hisao becomes involved in some aspect of macrobiotic teaching.

Reflections on Family

The family is the oldest and most enduring human institution. I have learned many things from my husband and children and from my parents, grandparents, brothers and sisters, and other relatives and ancestors. Though we have been separated by an ocean, we have kept up family ties. I thank God all my children are healthy. They all enjoy each other, keep in touch, and are practicing macrobiotics.

Since experimenting briefly in New York, I never used modern birth control methods. Over the years, I have come to see giving birth on a much bigger scale. It is really beyond the planning of the parents. The Order of Universe decides when each baby is born.

About twenty years ago, my husband started to check our children's birthdays to see if there was any pattern to them. He found that they all fell between his birthday and mine and on days and months in perfect harmony with our own. Our family was amazed at this discovery. From there we began to see the birth of each child as contributing to the whole family structure. In the case of an abortion, family balance automatically collapses because total order is violated. Also the spacing of the children follows a definite pattern. In Japan, my brothers and sisters were usually born about two years apart. My children arrived more logarithmically: one year, two years, four years, something like that.

When children are young, their problems are small. When they grow up and have their own families, their energy can be very harmonious and inspiring. But once quarrels between husband and wife begin, big problems arise. I'm sure all parents are concerned with the health and happiness of their children and their families. But as teachers and educators, my husband and I felt especially concerned. Over the years, Michio and I have given many seminars on man/woman relations and taught that separation and divorce are serious sicknesses.

In the Boston macrobiotic community, many couples separated, including some senior teachers and managers of our enterprises. It was always very sad. My husband and I counseled our young American friends. We encouraged them to remain together if possible, especially if they had children. Often the way of life, or way of eating, had become disorderly, and the husband or wife simply became too imbalanced. In many cases, a change in cooking—for example, less salt or more salt or variety—brought them back together again, and everyone was very happy.

In Japan the divorce rate is less than in America. Many times, when our children were growing up, my husband and I wished they could find Japanese mates. But they were not attracted to Japanese. I guess it is the destiny of our family to be international. In Japan, there is a proverb, "To marry, check the parents, not the children." After my own children grew up, several of them, as I have noted, began to have problems in their marriages. Three of them divorced or separated. In each case, our children's partner was a very nice person and also had studied with us. We miss them and are sorry they couldn't be together.

My children's family troubles have caused me a lot of self-reflection. I sometimes think as parents we spoiled them. Whatever they wanted to do, we accepted and supported them. In this respect, we are just following our parents who supported us without reservation. Marriage is really about the passage of human life. When we grew up, times were easy. Many of my children's marriage problems happened in 1986, a 5-Soil year according to traditional Nine Star Ki. Also, it was the year of Halley's Comet. As the year went by, I began to feel that the strong electromagnetic charge or influence of this comet as it passed by might be leading to confusion and disorder.

My husband is more hopeful. In talking over our children's situation, he always says, "Everything is going well. The right solution will come." He reminds me that whatever happens, including comets that come only once in a lifetime, is part of the Order of the Universe. We should be thankful for our difficulties.

Over the years, like most mothers, I have been strongly attached to my children. Their adversities have opened my eyes, and I have grown closer to my grandchildren as well as our friends' children. I feel the same about the young friends who have come to study and live with us. By the time we moved to Brookline, Lilly calculated that we had had about three hundred people stay with us in our different homes, not including our study houses or short-time guests. Since then, I'm sure the total has grown to at least a thousand. Every one of them is like one of the family, and my husband and I are always happy to hear news of them and their current activities.

I really admire the support that a traditional family structure provides. Sometimes we feel sorry for our children and our relatives. We have devoted so much time to our planetary family that we have not had so much time for them. But in one respect I am very happy. Our children normally call their friends family, and I think that is an important step in the spiritual development of humanity. My deepest wish is for all the children of the world to grow strong, be healthy, and enjoy peace. They are our life.

Relatives

After first coming to the United States, we lost touch with many of our relatives and friends in Japan. It has not been until recently that we have been able to resume communications with many of them. Of course, they had heard about our activities promoting health and diet. But until we were able to see and explain to them, it was hard to really understand what we were doing.

After World War II, Miyako, my eldest sister, returned from Manchuria with her husband and two children. He started to teach in Maki, the mountain village where I taught, for a couple of years. During the war, all Christian churches united to form the Japan Christian Association. After the war, individual sects came back into existence. My sister and brother-in-law moved to Tokyo and again became active in the Salvation Army. Her children, born in Manchuria on the Asian continent, had very strong constitutions in comparison to Japanese born in the islands. They were very yang like Seiji Ozawa, the director of the Boston Symphony Orchestra who was born in Manchuria during the war, and Toshiro Mifune, the actor, who was also born in China of Japanese parents. One of my nephews is now in real estate in Manhattan. I notice that he has a large head, is unusually strong, active and bold. My sister and her husband served for many years operating the church's rehabilitation center in Osaka. They are now retired.

My eldest brother, Makoto, took over Father's business after the war. But traditional silkscreening declined, and for many years he has operated a dry cleaning establishment. He married a woman from a Christian family near Matsue. They live in our family home in Yokota, taking care of our parents' and ancestors' graves. He and his wife brought up several children, and he has been very active in the Boy Scouts, like Father, and in local village politics.

Atsumi, my youngest sister, married after the war and moved to the next province. She has also raised an honest Christian family of three children and was active in her husband's business. He collected silk to send to distributors in Kyoto. Atsumi is now studying Noh drama and recently came to visit us at summer camp in the Berkshires. Her daughter, Mariko, came to study with us at our lovely retreat center in Becket and married one of our students.

Kyū, my next younger brother, graduated from the agricultural institute in Yokota after the war. As I mentioned in the chapter about our early days in New York, we invited him to help establish a gift shop in Greenwich Village. He took care of the merchandizing and inventory. Everyone was impressed with his earnestness and hard work. Later he became a merchandise warehouse manager of Takashimaya, the big department store we helped set up on Fifth Avenue. He married a lady from Hiroshima who had been introduced to him through the church at home. They had never met but

had exchanged photographs and letters. She came to New
York and they were married. Their marriage has been very
good, producing three children. They now live outside of
New York City and are making tofu, distributing Japanese
vegetables, and teaching farmers here how to grow burdock,
daikon, Chinese cabbage, and other vegetables. They are not
strictly macrobiotic but have been influenced by the teachings.

Junko, my second youngest sister, taught high school and
elementary school after graduating from teacher's college.
She married a fine Buddhist gentleman. I knew him at the
high school where I was teaching. He was young and had
just started teaching gymnastics. He later served as the principal of the high school in the region for many years. Recently
they retired and visited us in Brookline and have become
interested in macrobiotic agriculture.

When I was teaching in Maki, Yōko, my youngest sister,
was in first grade. She and our last brother, Masaru, came
to see me. I remember that they were just like kinder-
garteners. Later in New York, preparing for the opening of
Takashimaya and just before Phiya's birth, I invited her to
come and help us. She stayed with us in Queens and later got
a job with the Japan Travel Agency. After we moved to
Boston, she visited us many times. She eventually met and
married a young man working at Erewhon. His name was
Charles Kendall, and he was a very independent person.
Today they are living in western Massachusetts where they
make amazake, mochi, and other high quality macrobiotic
foods. Their company, Kendall Foods, is now supplying all of
New England and other parts of the United States with high
quality products.

Masaru, my youngest brother, went into the Merchant
Marine. His school had the biggest sailboat. After graduation,
he worked on a shipline out of Yokohama and crossed the
Pacific Ocean to Los Angeles and back. He had always dreamed
of being a good captain. In the old days, the captain was really
important to his ship. But nowadays, ships are controlled
by radar. He lost interest in sailing and came to New York

to stay with us. He studied Spanish and got a job with Japan Express, a big international cargo company. He worked out of Los Angeles for a long time, then moved to Miami, and is now managing the office in New Jersey. He is very quiet and active. He married a classmate, a girl I used to know from a nearby town. They have two sons.

Michio's parents visited us in Cambridge shortly after we moved to the Boston area. He was always concerned that his parents might disapprove of his activities and would ask him to come home. They had always wanted him to become a government leader, ambassador, or successful diplomat. After staying in our house for several weeks, they told him that they had decided to become his students. Michio was stunned, but happy. Afterward, he said he knew he could change the whole world because changing parents is the hardest thing of all.

My husband has spoken and written a great deal about his mother, Teru, and the influence that she has had on his life. She was very active socially. She served as a judge for the Tokyo Family Court for many years. She was strong and creative—very yang. Michio has that side too. George Ohsawa met Michio's parents after he came to the United States. Ordinary scholars saw George Ohsawa as strange and didn't really understand macrobiotics. George Ohsawa said when he met Michio's parents, he really trusted Michio. He was particularly struck by his mother. Her character was very strong. He said she always went in front, while her husband supported her. After we moved to Brookline, she passed away in Japan.

Michio's brother came to see us for the first time in Brookline. He works for JETRO, the Japanese External Trade Organization. He was stationed in Houston, Seoul, Korea, and other places before returning to Tokyo to take care of his parents. He and his wife have four children, and we always see them when we visit Japan.

After Michio's mother died, his father accompanied us on a trip to Europe. He had been a history teacher and school principal for most of his life. He specialized in European history and had written the sections on the Renaissance for many Japanese history books. In London he spent a long time looking at the old Roman gate to the city. He delighted in seeing ancient ruins and artifacts reflecting contact between different cultures. But his biggest joy was in Florence. Several years earlier, he had visited Italy on a group tour. There was a tour guide, but Michio's father knew so much more that soon he was asked to take over. All the travelers were very happy.

Before setting out in Florence, Keizo knew by heart the names of all the streets, castles, churches, houses, rivers, and mountains. For him, seeing Giotto's bell tower, the Palazzo Vecchio, or the spires of Santa Croce was like being reunited with a lost lover. His favorite site was the great Cathedral in the center of the city. It houses a famous statue of David by Michelangelo. Michio's father was very healthy and had never been absent a day in over forty years' teaching. But now he was in his eighties, and we were concerned that he not overexert himself. The way he scampered up the steep stairway inside the Cathedral, it was all Michio and Norio could do to keep up with him. At the top, they walked around Brunelleschi's big dome and examined the marvelous murals that covered the ceiling. Then they went outside on the roof of the Cathedral, which had a breathtaking view of all Florence. Michio's father spent hours up there, observing the winding curves of the Arno River and the city spread out before him. He loved Dante, Beatrice, Leonardo, Savaranola, and the other great men and women who had lived in Florence and knew all the streets and bridges they had once walked.

Several hundred macrobiotic friends came to our seminars, and Michio's father also spoke. After our trip to Europe, Keizo said that he was more convinced than before that Michio was right to have followed his own destiny.

While traveling together, I saw that Michio was very similar to his father. Both father and son were very patient and humble. The elder Kushi never said to his children or grandchildren "do this or do that." He was very respectful. During his retirement, he researched the family history and made a beautiful family tree. He traced his ancestors back thousands of years to Afghanistan, India, and Africa. There was an old family proverb, "The treasure of the Kushi family lies in the east." From Japan, America lies east, so perhaps his son's journey and settling here are a part of that ancient prophecy.

13: Dancing on an Empty Stage

"A bit of earth will make the mountain higher, a
drop of water makes the ocean deeper."

—Kōbō Daishi

OVER THE YEARS, we have met many friends who are
very talented. After becoming macrobiotic, they found
that their painting, singing, or writing improved.
After we moved to Boston, one of the women I admired most
was Gloria Swanson. As a student in college, I had seen movies
of her and Charlie Chaplain. Then in the 1950s, I saw *Sunset
Boulevard*. She had been eating natural foods for many years
before she became involved in macrobiotic activities. In
the *East West Journal*, she wrote an article, "I Am Still
a Woman," telling how she healed herself of a uterine tumor
with proper diet. Her gynecologist wanted her to have immediate surgery and was shocked when she got up from his
examination table and walked out of the door.

We first met Gloria through William Dufty, who had become macrobiotic after meeting George Ohsawa in Paris. She
and Bill had their marriage ceremony in our home in Brookline. Gloria was a very unique, unusual person. She and her
husband always brought along their own food and a lot of
cookware on their travels. One time they came to Boston to
see us. Gloria.was in her seventies and still radiant. A friend
asked her how she managed to keep her skin and face so
beautiful. She showed us a small cotton hand towel in her
handbag. She kept it wrapped in plastic.

"This is my secret," she said.

She explained that she wiped her face and skin with it
whenever she had time. She said she put nothing on her face,
just scrubbed it with the rough towel.

One time Gloria and Bill visited Japan with us. She enjoyed the Far East very much, but it took some adjusting for her. We visited Mount Koya, an ancient Buddhist pilgrimage site, and stayed in traditional accommodations in a temple. The air was exhilarating and the landscaping exquisite. There were bright red and purple azaleas everywhere, rows of yellow dandelions, and meditative ponds with wonderfully shaped rocks and stones. The next morning I asked Gloria if she had slept well in this lovely environment. She said she had trouble sleeping because of the sound of the bullfrogs in the pond.

She also had trouble with the Japanese style toilets and the smell of the hot springs, but she enjoyed the food very much. The Japanese people know her from her movies, especially those who are my age or older. They recognized and followed her wherever she went, just as people do in the United States. She was very surprised.

In New York, Gloria lived in a beautiful apartment. She was a talented sculptor and painter as well as actress. I was very impressed with the way she held flowers and handled ordinary, everyday things gracefully and without any special effort. She had beautiful posture and was very careful in the way she took things when eating. We grew very close.

Bill Dufty is one of the happiest, most amazing friends we have. Many people know him from his books, *You Are All Sanpaku* and *Sugar Blues*. In person, he is extraordinary. He always speaks his mind. He doesn't care what other people think. He is a free man. Sometimes his words give a shock to us too. But that is his way to awaken people. In traveling, I noticed that he is also very free. In Japan, he didn't mind curling up in the corner of the street to take a nap. From the beginning of our macrobiotic activity in Boston, he has given us suggestions. Sometimes we couldn't follow his advice. It was a pity because he usually was right. At conferences and seminars, Bill is a strong speaker, and his talks always have a big impact. People enjoy his wry sense of humor. He also enjoys dancing, and at macrobiotic parties, we like to dance together.

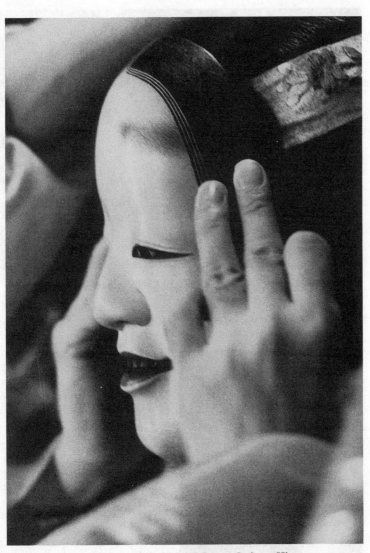

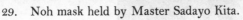

29. Noh mask held by Master Sadayo Kita.

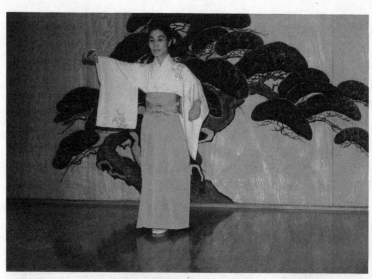

30. *Above*, Aveline performing Noh dance in Los Angeles, 1971.

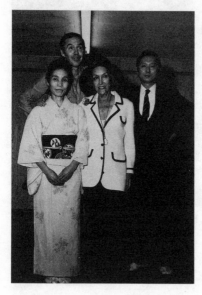

31.
Aveline with Bill Dufty,
Gloria Swanson, and Master
Kita.

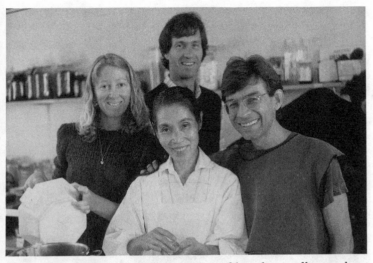

32. Like thousands of macrobiotic cooking classes all over the world, this one ended in smiles.

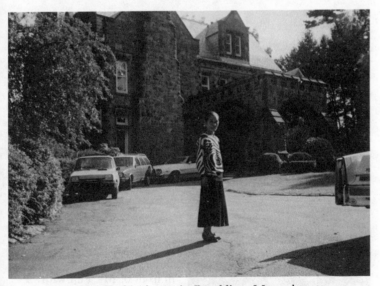

33. The Kushis' house in Brookline, Massachusetts.

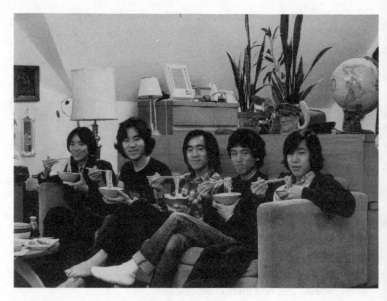

34.
Above, the five Kushi children enjoying noodles: Lilly, Norio, Haruo, Phiya, and Hisao.

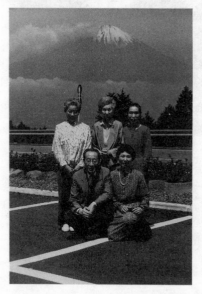

35.
In front of Mt. Fuji with Michio, Lima Ohsawa (top center) and two macrobiotic friends from Japan.

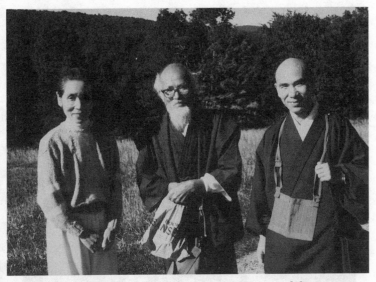

36. Aveline at Kushi Institute in Becket with natural farmer
Masanobu Fukuoka and Esoteric Buddhist priest Rev. Tanaka.

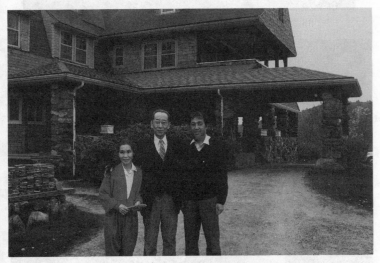

37. In front of the main house at the Kushi Institute in Becket with
Kazuhiro Irie, a Japanese friend.

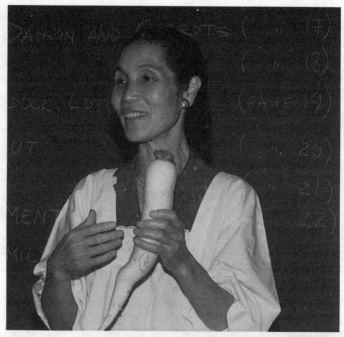

38. Demonstrating daikon at a cooking class.

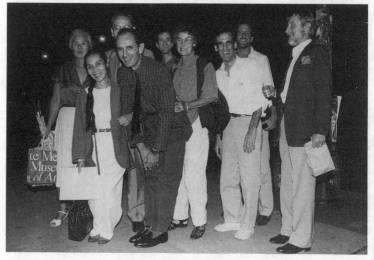

39. With Anthony Muto, Dr. Martha C. Cottrell, and other macrobiotic teachers in New York after an AIDS seminar.

279

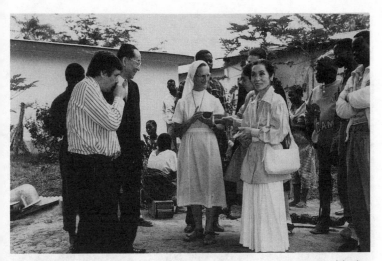

40. On a visit to Africa in 1987, the Kushis started a macrobiotic educational campaign to prevent AIDS. *Above*, discussing organic farming with Sister Theresa and associates in the Congo.

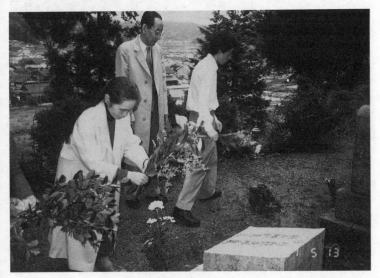

41. The Kushis and their son Phiya at the graves of Aveline's parents on a mountainside overlooking Yokota.

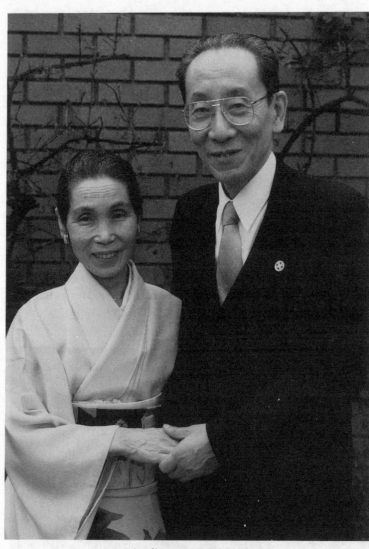

42. Aveline and Michio Kushi.

John Denver became a good friend in the early 1980s. The first time we went to see him in Colorado, one of the girls working at the Kushi Foundation was so excited, she kept exclaiming, "John Denver wants to see Michio!" We had never heard of John Denver. My daughter asked me to come up to her room. She had all his music. I went up immediately and listened to some songs from *Country Roads*, his album about West Virginia. I liked them very much. In Colorado, John came to my cooking classes. I was impressed with his humble spirit. John recognized right away that cooking was a supreme art. He later said that after becoming macrobiotic, he was able to sing like a bird.

In Boston, John later gave a benefit concert for the Kushi Foundation. We met him on numerous occasions, and he joined our board of directors. He asked Michio and me to serve on Windstar, his foundation in Aspen devoted to ecological harmony, renewable energy, and other aspects of natural living. We were very honored by his invitation and enjoyed visiting his lovely home.

In New England or New York, we always try to attend John Denver's concerts when he is performing. He now represents macrobiotics all over the world with his songs. Michio and I feel his spirit reflects the true heart of the American land. His warm, strong, beautiful energy radiates through his songs. He is also very active in cross-cultural exchanges and peace education in this country, the Soviet Union, and China. Whether you see him in person or just listen to his records, John Denver conveys a happy, healthy feeling.

One time, on a trip to see John in Colorado, I was met at the airport by Robert Fulton! He was our first student, friend, and associate from the days in Queens, Martha's Vineyard, and Cambridge. We had not been in touch for over twenty years. He picked me up in a big Cadillac and explained that he had become a movie producer. It seemed like just yesterday that we were together on Cape Cod.

The Tea Ceremony

The best music, painting, or sculpture makes you healthy, happy, and whole just by listening to it or seeing it. That is my definition of art. Over the years, I have devoted myself to several artistic pursuits besides cooking.

The Tea Ceremony is a traditional aspect of Far Eastern culture. In an introduction to the classic *The Book of Tea*, Tenshin Okakura traced the little known impact of tea-drinking on the West. Of course, in Boston, home of the Boston Tea Party, we know the influence very well. He observed, "East meets West in a cup of tea." When I was in college, it was common to study the Tea Ceremony and flower arrangement. The first two years I studied tea—the style of the Omote-senke school—and the third and fourth years, I studied flowers.

In New York I became very friendly with a Japanese Tea Ceremony master who started a Tea Ceremony school. I was one of his original students and also studied later in Los Angeles. In Boston, there was an old Japanese teahouse stored in a warehouse. The teahouse had not been used for many years. George Matson, the director of the Matson Academy of Karate where George Ohsawa and Michio gave their first lecture in Boston, talked the authorities into moving it to his academy. Later it was moved to the Children's Museum in Jamaica Plain, and I sometimes taught the Tea Ceremony there after moving to Cambridge. From Japan, Michio's parents sent us a beautiful tea set. I also demonstrated the Tea Ceremony at cultural exchange gatherings sponsored by the Japan Society. I used to carry everything in a big padded suitcase. Sometimes a macrobiotic friend would help me drive and carry it to the demonstration. Besides cooking classes, I also taught the Tea Ceremony to macrobiotic friends. Traditionally, the green tea powder used in the ceremony has a very bitter taste. It is usually served with sweets. Today in Japan, they're using sugar. I hope they change back to a natural sweetener. I often gave demonstrations using only tea.

The essence of the Tea Ceremony is appreciation of a cup

of tea and beautiful movement. The tea maker picks up implements and puts them down in a certain way. The ritual appears deceptively simple. But it takes long years of study and concentration to master. In the hands of a master, the Tea Ceremony is a symphony of yang and yin—motion and rest. The tea maker and the person or persons served become one. If the ceremony is performed properly, they glimpse or experience the world of infinity.

In addition to taking us to the realm of higher consciousness, the Tea Ceremony is very practical. It teaches us how to use ordinary, everyday things very efficiently and economically. The macrobiotic kitchen is nothing but the Tea Ceremony on a larger scale. At home, we can create and convey the same serene quality of consciousness in the foods we prepare. By carefully putting all our energy into whatever we are doing, we produce something harmonious, balanced, and beautiful. This includes cutting vegetables, pouring spring water, and tending the fire. Each step contributes to the vibration and energy of the whole. The quality of our meals is a reflection of our mind and spirit, our health and vitality. Using the same ingredients, we can produce a calm, peaceful effect on those who eat our food, or we can create disorder. True cooking is meditation in action. We become aware of our breathing. We become one with our environment. A simple cup of tea or bowl of brown rice can elevate our spirit, reconcile man and woman, and unify East and West. This is the heart of macrobiotic cooking.

Futons and Fabrics

Sewing and making clothes are another traditional art I have enjoyed over the years. In New York, I made clothing for my children, sleeping kimonos for my husband, and kimonos and dresses for myself. As a child, I had helped my father in the silkscreen workshop and became nostalgic for natural fabrics. One of my joys in New York was going to remnant stores to pick up good quality, but inexpensive cottons, silks, and wools.

Day and night, I would sit at my sewing machine when I wasn't cooking or cleaning. Making clothes became my hobby and vacation. I was especially busy making clothes during pregnancies. I got very yang at these times, and it was not easy to sleep. I also took up embroidery and crocheting. I once crocheted a cotton carpet which my family enjoyed very much.

In Boston, I gave classes on making kimonos. Many times I gave kimonos as gifts. I also made shoulder bags like I used in school and college. In Cambridge, I went to an upholstery store, and they gave me some remnants free. I was excited and made many beautiful shoulder bags. Many of my kimonos and shoulder bags were sold at Erewhon.

I also taught how to make futons—traditional Japanese mattresses—and *zabuton* meditation cushions. In Los Angeles, I found beautiful cotton batting just as in Japan. In Hollywood, at the house on Franklin Street, I made a futon instead of a bed. It was the first futon I had to sleep on in America. My mother had made futons, so I knew the technique. In L.A.'s Japan Town, I found some dried silk worm nests. Threads from this source are traditionally used to sew the cover on the batting. Other thread doesn't hold up as well. I bought the shop's whole supply and made sixty futons. Thirty of them were for people at our study house.

After returning to Boston, I ordered cotton batting and gave my first futon-making class. Unfortunately, the cotton was rough, and we couldn't get silk worm thread. I also found that it was necessary to make futons slightly different for Americans than for Japanese. In Japan, houses are very small. There are are no bedrooms. The same room is used for everything. At night, after dinner and evening conversation, futons will be laid on the floor. In the morning, they will be folded up and put on a closet shelf out of the way. The only futon that stays out all the time is called a "million-year bed." It is for long-time sick people or those about to journey to the next world. In Japan, some people sleep directly on wood. There is a wafer-thin futon known as the *senbei* or flat futon. It is

the cheapest type. Futons in Japan today are softer, richer,
and lacier in comparison, but they are made with synthetic
materials.

Compared to Japan, houses here are much bigger. People
have their own bedrooms. Also, people here are not used to
sitting or sleeping on the floor. The floors themselves are
made of hardwood or covered with carpet. In Japan, floors
are cushioned with thick tatami straw mats. I saw right
away that Americans were not comfortable sleeping on thin
futons. We started making heavier ones. They were too
thick to fold up, but they could be rolled. In Japan we
sometimes made silk coverings for futons from old kimonos,
but usually we used cotton. Mother made lovely tie-dye
designs. In America we used heavier sailcloth. In our classes,
we would all sew with big needles. It was like sewing canvas.

My students and I had enjoyable times sewing together.
We would laugh, and I told stories of how futons are traditionally made in Japan. Once a year, Mother would take off
all the futon covers and wash them. Japan is very humid, so
we traditionally did this on the hottest day of the summer, at
the end of July. The cotton batting would then be sent to a
mill. There it would be compressed and reconstituted for use.
In all the rice fields, mothers and daughters would be outside
busy at work over rows of futons. I helped many times.

I also showed my students how to take care of natural
fabrics. I was surprised that young women and girls here
didn't know the first thing about washing and protecting their
clothing and bedding. We learned these things in elementary
school. Several ladies who studied with me started the first
futon companies in America. Later, elegant wooden frames and
other furniture were added. Even with thick futons, Americans still preferred to sleep off the floor.

Noh Drama

In Los Angeles, I started studying Noh, the classical drama
of Japan. I had always loved dancing and acting. In fourth

grade, a small theater was built in Yokota. Father made
a stage curtain, drapery, and scenery for it, and I helped draw
the mountains and rivers in the background. In college, I
studied ballet and waltz but not traditional Japanese dance.
Noh stories were all familiar to me as literature, and sometimes they would show up in a movie, but until I found a Noh
teacher on the West Coast, I never had a chance to study Noh
performance for myself. Until I actually saw the stories en-
acted and heard the singing that accompanied them, I could
not fully appreciate this wonderful way of life.

In Los Angeles, I was busy taking care of my son, running
a study house, giving cooking classes, and setting up Erewhon-
L.A., but I became passionately devoted to Noh. My teacher
was a top master. He came over to the States in the summer.
We met in a small theater in Japan Town. There were thirty
members in the group. They were mostly middle aged or
older, including several retired people. I was impressed with
the many types of people in my classes. Some of them had
been put in concentration camps in New Mexico or Arizona
during World War II. The land at that time was a desert.
The Japanese-Americans watered it, grew things, and turned
it green. Mr. Sasaki, the landscape architect at Harvard from
whom we bought land in Ashburnham, Massachusetts, for
our East West Foundation rural community, had also been in
a camp as a child. That's where he developed his interest
in landscaping. In the camp, the people taught each other
traditional arts and ways of living. This Noh drama group
was organized there. They had since moved to Los Angeles
and had been singing, dancing, and performing together for
many years.

Master Sadayo Kita, our teacher, taught us privately, one
by one. Every day, we received instruction in singing and
dancing. Each time we used a different text. In addition to
my own lessons, I watched the other students, from morning
to night if I could.

Mr. Kita joked about my earnestness, "I never saw such
a crazy student in my life."

I learned quickly and soon he instructed me in advanced dancing. It was very easy to pick up. There is a proverb: "Dancing takes three years to master, singing seven years." I made tape-recordings of the singing, but never really perfected it.

Noh is traditionally performed by members of the same family. In Japan, the tradition has been passed down in certain families now for thirteen or fourteen generations. Mr. Kita's ancestors were members of a samurai family who started their school a little later, in the sixteen century. His grandfather, Roppeita Kita, was considered Japan's greatest recent Noh master, and he himself has been named a Priceless Cultural Treasure by the government today.

Mr. Kita first performed at age six. The actors practice all the time. Some roles, however, are not allowed to be performed before age sixty. It is common for Noh singers and dancers to still be active at age eighty or ninety. I noticed while practicing that the soul of the drama was very different when older people directed or participated in it.

Noh originated in Izumo, my province, "the ancient home of the gods." Performance and repertory go back to the early fifteenth century when country pantomime was transformed into a courtly art. The rural theater appears to have some connection with the rice festival. The purpose of the first performances may have been to reap the best harvests. Later, Zen became influenced by or associated with Noh, though it is not directly connected. Okuni, one of the founders of Noh, was a lady. However, customarily Noh is performed only by men. The costumes are so heavy that the actors must be very strong. Also during pregnancy and menstruation, women could not always go on stage. After World War II, that began to change. Now there are a few ladies in Japan performing Noh.

Many Noh stories are about the spiritual world. Ghosts come back to earth to talk. Spirits and demons appear and disappear on stage, dancing and telling stories. Samurai are also frequently subjects of Noh tales. They are vanquished soldiers mostly or the souls of samurai that have been slain on the battlefield. In only one or two Noh stories are they victorious. The stories are drawn from *The Tale of Genji*, *The Tale of the Heike*, and other classics. The audiences already know the outcome, so what is important is the characterization and depth of feeling conveyed by the actors.

Traditionally, if the Noh actor made a mistake, he committed *hara-kiri*. Mr. Kita tried to change the form and content of some of the performances, but found the old pattern best. He says that after age ninety, a performer may be qualified to alter things if he likes. Performances are never stopped for any reason, even if an actor suffers a heart attack. When that happens, there is always someone behind the stage who knows his lines and will come in to take over.

Until the Meiji era, Noh was performed only in shrines or temples and before the lords and nobles During the Tokugawa era, which lasted for nearly three centuries, the Kita family was one of five troupes chosen by the shōgun to perform on high ceremonial occasions of state. Farmers or villagers were not allowed to watch or take part. The people's theater, or Kabuki, developed as a result. Kabuki is very different from Noh. Noh is slow, meditative. The actions are very refined. Kabuki is fast, emotional. Movements are exaggerated. In Kabuki there is a long walkway to the stage. People in the audience customarily dine from beautiful lunchboxes or drink sake. They call out to their favorite actors and throw towels on stage. Noh is much more formal. Performers never bow when they come on stage. Traditionally, there is complete silence among the audience. Even after the performers finish, the audience refrains from clapping. Noh leaves a beautiful vibration on stage that clapping destroys. But that too has changed in the present day, and some audiences applaud loudly.

Because of its strong connection with the world of spirit, Noh has been banned from Mount Koya, the Buddhist pilgrimage center. When it was performed there in the past, too many spirits and wandering souls would gather, bringing thunderstorms and lightening and frightening the monks and pilgrims. During World War II, the government stopped almost all entertainment throughout Japan. My teacher recalls performing at this time in empty shrines and temples. He told me they sang and danced for the gods.

In Boston, I set up a small Noh academy, the Kita Noh Institute of America. We rented space in the building next to Arlington Street Church (later used for the East West Foundation offices). I applied for a grant from the Japan Foundation and invited Mr. Kita to come and teach during the summers. It was one of the first times Noh had been performed or taught in Boston. Many people attended, including drama and dance teachers from around New England. We held performances at Andover, Wellesley, Harvard, Boston University, and many theaters. The first two years, Mr. Kita came alone. Later the entire troupe of eleven actors came and performed at the New England Life Center and John Hancock Hall. The performances included *Tomoe*, a battlefield dance done in full costume about the wife of Kiso Yoshinaka, one of Japan's most famous warriors. The ghost of Tomoe, performed by Mr. Kita, returns to the battlefield many years later and tells a traveling priest the story of how she fought alongside her husband and how he was killed. In *Uto*, Mr. Kita assumed the role of the spirit of a hunter who is suffering in the afterlife because of having killed birds.

From practicing and observing on stage, I noticed that the Noh mask is the essence of the performance. The angle at which the mask is worn expresses emotions. A slightly lifted mask indicates happiness. A mask that is held downward shows sadness. Mr. Kita always carried his own masks. When we went anywhere by car or plane, he never allowed anyone else to handle them. Generally the stages where we performed were dirty and the dressing rooms unclean. To protect the costumes and masks, I took heavy construction paper everywhere we went. I would dust the room and then tape the construction paper down from corner to corner. Then Mr. Kita would start to dress. The other members of the troupe were also very conscientious. I observed they were careful about eating. Although they were not macrobiotic, they didn't take cold foods before a performance. Nor would they eat overly relaxing foods like eggplant or rich foods like tempura. None of the actors was fat. All seemed moderate and balanced. They also meditated before a performance as was customary.

One time we helped with *Madame Butterfly*, which was being performed by the Boston Opera Company. One of our member's wives was a professional dresser and had been asked to help prepare the beautiful bridal kimono for that production. We got a good look at what it was like behind stage at a big American theater. We were shocked at the difference. Though expensive in cost, the costumes were made of the cheapest materials and thrown away at the end of the production. In Japan, it can take ten years to make one robe. The costumes we were using had been made a hundred years ago and were handed down lovingly from father to son. The opera stage was dirty. The costume they borrowed from us was returned soiled. The kimono we lent was torn and unusable. I enjoyed *Madame Butterfly* very much and met many fine actors and actresses. But the approach was so completely different.

In Noh, the dressing room is called the mirror room. After putting on his costume, the Noh master puts on his mask in front of the mirror and watches himself. He has to become the main character. This process is also very much a meditation. Different masks are used: samurai, ladies, demons, animals. The masks themselves don't move. Beautiful feelings are expressed by the actors' movements. Mask making is traditionally one of the highest arts. In college, I enjoyed the story of Izuno Yashaō, a famous sculptor and mask maker. He was ordered to make the mask of an early, feared shōgun. An image of death appeared on the mask he made and he destroyed it. He made another mask. Again he didn't like it and destroyed it. The shōgun became impatient and sent a servant to pick it up. Izuno promised to have it ready soon. But again he destroyed it, although he knew the heavy consequences of disobeying the shōgun. Then a special messenger came with news that the shōgun had been assassinated. Izuno rejoiced. His prophecy had come true.

Today Noh is more popular in Japan than in the past. Now it can be seen on TV. Noh combines the essence of drama, singing, meditation, and spiritual development. I would love to study it more. It is a wonderful bridge between cultures. In Japan, Noh masters and traditional costume and mask makers are venerated. Many countries have traditions like this in music, art, and literature. They are nourishment for the spirit. My dream is that macrobiotic friends and families around the world will preserve these cultural treasures for the enjoyment of future generations just as they are saving traditional grains, beans, and seeds.

Chanting and Meditation

On my second visit to Japan, I had a remarkable experience. I was visiting my family home in Yokota and sitting by the *kotatsu*. This is the low, heated, recessed table in the front room that is used for dining, conversation, and keeping warm. I had just arrived from Osaka to visit my relatives and had only two days to stay because of our busy schedule. As I was sitting there, I suddenly lost all sense of time and space.

I lost consciousness and felt transported to the realm of eternity. I had never experienced such a feeling. I had many deep, joyful experiences in the mountains and traveling around the world, but this was different. I forgot the past and present. Even my thoughts of family, husband, and children all disappeared.

I don't know how long I remained in that state. Perhaps ten minutes. When I regained ordinary consciousness, I was shocked. I realized that I probably had the experience because I was back home in the village of my birth. It was also the same room where I was sick so many years before and had written my poems of "Clouds Passing By." I knew that I always had a peaceful mountain village to go home to. I felt sorry for my children and friends who did not have a place like this to return to. In Tokyo, New York, Boston, or other modern cities around the world, it is very hard to find a place of such unsurpassed natural beauty.

I thought back and remembered that Buddha had lived about eighty or ninety years. He walked from village to village around India, finally returning in the direction of his birthplace. According to tradition, he passed into nirvana facing his homeland.

On this trip to Japan, I had been searching for a teacher to help me understand Buddhism. As I grew older, I began to feel that I should do some exercises for my mental and spiritual development. I had been reading some books on Shingon, an esoteric school of Buddhism that is well known in Japan and has a long tradition. One day in Munich, Germany, where we were giving a seminar, I met a young Japanese tourist in our hotel. I chatted with him and found that the author of the book I was reading was his teacher. I wanted to meet him. A few months later, on this visit to Japan, I made an appointment. I really didn't care for his book and was disappointed in his center. They were presenting the teachings not in the traditional way but in a more popular style.

My experience of God or infinity in Yokota was spontaneous and short-lived. I hoped that by finding a meditation teacher I could control and polish my awareness. On the same trip, I visited Koyasan, the historic Buddhist mountain community two hours' train ride south of Osaka. Here, in the misty clouds and among lofty pine trees that reach up to the heavens, are nestled nearly "a hundred hundred" Buddhist temples. Many of them date to the eighth century when Kōbō Daishi, the founder of Esoteric Buddhism, lived. On Mount Koya, I read another book and loved it. I studied on my own back home in Boston and then learned that Rev. Jyomyo Tanaka, a Shingon priest, had arrived in New York. I contacted him and started to study. He had only five or six students. On weekends, I would drive from Brookline to New York. Sometimes one or two friends accompanied me. We met in a small apartment in Greenwich Village. I usually drove home the same day.

Rev. Tanaka used Kōbō Daishi's text. Ordinarily it is not shown to ordinary people or women, but in coming to America, Esoteric Buddhism, like Zen Buddhism and other Far Eastern teachings, underwent significant changes. The practice took two hours each morning and included prayer, chanting, bells, incense, and meditation. Every day, for a hundred days, I would get up early and perform the ritual. It required a lot of concentration.

During his lifetime, Kōbō Daishi was known as Kukai, which means "Sky and Sea." The essence of his teaching is known as "Soku shinjō butsu." By this is meant that we are already enlightened. Kukai taught that everyone already has Buddha nature or is a child of God. We don't need to die or go to the next world. In Sanskrit, we learned to chant sutras or verses and visualize the different wisdom beings. There are chants for the Medicine Buddha, the Children's Buddha, the Sun Buddha, and many others. The mantra—or sound itself—is considered Buddha or God. By chanting, performing gestures with the hands, and contemplating the different aspects of wisdom, we realize our Buddhahood—our original, clear, free, natural mind.

In his lectures, my husband was teaching heaven and earth's energy. He said that everything is created by vibration. By studying meditation, we can really feel and catch that vibration. After chanting, I could understand Noh drama better. My breathing improved. I became happier, more relaxed, generally brighter, and more cheerful.

In the beginning, it was very difficult to meditate. But once I memorized the chants and learned the basic form, so many things started happening. I came to see meditation as a way of receiving energy. It is like recharging your battery. When I get tired, now I know how to meditate, and real *ki*, or electromagnetic energy, from the universe, comes in. My breathing also improved. I had always heard that *sennin*—free men—breathed from the feet, but I had never experienced it before for myself. Through my practice, that kind of deep breathing came naturally. My whole circulation became peaceful and quiet.

Through meditation, we can direct our energy or consciousness and heal many things. I found that I could control my eating for the first time. In recent years, I have eaten too many wonderful desserts at Open Sesame and other macrobiotic restaurants and too much food in general. I could never resist. After meditation, I could automatically control the volume of food, including rich dishes and delicious desserts, that I ate.

Many angles of teaching came together as a result of learning how to meditate. All principles and laws we study are nothing but ways to understand God, the universe, and ourselves and prepare for the next world. Everyone's destiny is death, or birth into the spiritual world. That is now really clear to me.

Another thing I noticed was my interest in books and movies. Like my husband, I always loved to read. I never got tired of classical novels. I used to weep over books and cry at the movies. I still enjoy these forms of study and relaxation, but I've found that I don't do them as much as before. Maybe I've just become more selective.

Overall, my daily practice has left me feeling brighter, steadier, and less worried. I still have very far to go. My husband always says he has no desires of his own. He simply waits for people to ask for his help. On the other hand, I have been too pushy. As at the Maison Ignoramus, when I reached for the axe, I have gained a reputation in Boston for strong, spontaneous action. I am always setting up businesses and enterprises, renting offices, looking at real estate, promoting seminars, and bringing people together for various activities. True to my wild boar nature, I've always plunged straight ahead, changing direction countless times. This pattern has begun to change, I think, as I've grown older. I feel I've gradually matured and am more accepting of others. Where I could only see one view before, now I see several. Perhaps my husband is also changing and moving in the other direction. Recently, he has devoted more and more energy again to the problem of war and peace in the nuclear age. He has also taken the initiative to start spiritual training seminars at our new retreat center in western Massachusetts.

One of the nice things about my studying Buddhist meditation was that it led Rev. Tanaka to study macrobiotics. After changing his way of eating, he found that the essense of Buddha's teachings was "shojin ryori" or the supreme art of cooking. That traditional way of eating has been lost in many Buddhist temples in the Far East. In Japan, priests and monks today eat meat and fish. But the shortest way to understand the teachings and achieve the goal of meditation is to eat well. Rev. Tanaka is now a regular teacher at our summer camp and participates in macrobiotic activities around the country.

Many friends have rediscovered their religious roots after becoming macrobiotic and have found that they are able to be better Christians, Jews, Moslems, Hindus, or Buddhists. Macrobiotics is the thread that unifies all religions, philosophies, and traditional ways of life. Though I was born a Christian, I feel at home in all churches, temples, and houses of worship. As people's health and judgment are restored through balanced food and reflection, religious wars and conflicts will become a thing of the past. The world of the future will see all faiths as expressions of the one Living God.

14: Planting the Seeds of Peace

> "It has never been possible to produce a delicious
> dish out of just one flavor or a beautiful melody out
> of one tone."   —Kōbō Daishi

THE ROAD to Becket winds several miles over a slowly
rising mountain. The forest is thick with foliage and
wildlife. If you are keen, you can sometimes see a deer
and its fawn crossing a meadow or field. In the mornings,
there is dew or a hint of frost on the ground. In the evenings,
the rays of the setting sun bathe the surrounding peaks and
lakes in a shower of crimson light. The road emerges in a
beautiful valley. With its small cluster of white-steepled
churches and frame houses, Becket Center is a sleepy New
England hamlet. About a half-mile up from the general store,
a dirt road branches off to the right. It leads through the
woods to a former Franciscan monastery.

In recent years, the abbey in Becket has become a second
hub of our educational activities. My husband and I constantly
go back and forth between the city and the country. Our teaching center in the Berkshires is located on six hundred acres of
woodland. The main house was originally constructed by a
wealthy banker as a hunting lodge. It is made in the Flemish
style of stone and timbers imported from Europe and includes
a large paneled dining room, living room with fireplace, and
ten upstairs bedrooms. Next door is a dormitory built by the
Catholic fathers. It includes accommodations for about thirty
people, a library, a refectory, and a beautiful chapel.

In the late 1970s, macrobiotics entered a new phase. For
a long time we had dreamed of expanding our educational
activities. Until then, our classes had been informal. Our staff

was volunteer. We met at homes, study houses, or churches. No degrees or certificates were granted. A natural community of learning developed, based on experience and higher judgment.

Among ourselves, we did not need the trappings of formal education. However, as the public became more attracted to our way of life, we needed to develop qualified teachers, counselors, and cooks. This became particularly important after our drive to free society from heart disease and cancer. Many of those who suffer with these problems and other degenerative disorders and their families came to us for guidance. It was essential that they receive proper advice and cooking. By now there were thousands of people around the world who had studied with us. Their understanding and practice varied considerably. Many were now teaching macrobiotics themselves, or combining it with various other approaches. For a serious illness such as the terminal stage of cancer, improper advice or cooking could be a matter of life and death.

In 1979, we started the Michio Kushi Institute for One Peaceful World. The first Kushi Institute was opened in London by Bill Tara. British currency was low, and it was expensive for some European friends to travel to America and study with us. The main center opened in Boston the following year. We looked at many places for a site and ended up in a converted warehouse in Brookline Village. Located at 17 Station Street across from the trolley stop into Boston, the building housed artists' and potters' studios. The Kushi Institute occupied three large rooms on the third floor. Two of them were made into classrooms and one was used for administration. On the second floor, a kitchen with an old cast-iron stove was remodeled for our cooking classes. The *East West Journal* later moved into the other studio on the third floor, and the East West Foundation set up counseling offices on the second floor. For the first time, all of our educational and publishing activities were united under one roof.

The Kushi Institute was in walking distance of many friends

who lived in Brookline Village and Jamaica Plain. My own
family now was living in a lovely house on Buckminster
Road, about a mile from the village. The Village Natural
Foods Store soon opened on Washington Street, around the
corner from the Kushi Institute. It was later taken over by
Erewhon. Nearby, on Route 9, Open Sesame Restaurant
started serving delicious macrobiotic food. Horai-San Gift
Shop opened next to the food store and carried a complete
line of macrobiotic books and cookware. Further out extended
the network of study houses. By now, we no longer took
an active role in their affairs. The Boston macrobiotic community, centered on Erewhon, was economically self-sufficient
enough to operate their own accommodations. Even after
Erewhon failed, most of the macrobiotic workforce was ab-
sorbed in other businesses and enterprises run by macrobiotic
people.

In Boston, we had enough experienced teachers to set up
a curriculum at the new Kushi Institute. Helping us from the
beginning was Shizuko Yamamoto. Shizuko grew up in Tokyo
and stayed single. She studied with George Ohsawa and became skilled in shiatsu. Shiatsu is the traditional acupressure
massage of the Far East. After George passed away, she came
to America and settled in New York. Shizuko and I became
close friends. She has a strong constitution and is very yang.
In New York, she put her whole personal effort into keeping
a macrobiotic center there active. Living in New York is very
intense. As in Paris, macrobiotic leaders and organizations
come and go quickly. For nearly twenty years now, Shizuko
has been the Pole Star of macrobiotic activities in Manhattan.
Many friends have studied with her. She comes regularly to
Boston, where she has taken charge of our shiatsu studies at
the Institute and summer camp.

Besides shiatsu, we offered basic studies in the Order of
the Universe, visual diagnosis, macrobiotic health and physical
and mental care, and macrobiotic cooking. Our first class of
students numbered seventeen. Only three of them were Americans. The rest came from all over the world, including Brazil,

Greece, Italy, Spain, Switzerland, Germany, France, and
Portugal. Caroline Heidenry and Olivia Oredsen, two devoted
young ladies who at that time had studied with us for about
ten years, served as first directors. Later, Bill Tara came back
from London and took charge of overall management. Across
the hall, Sherman Goldman and Alex Jack edited the *East
West Journal* and focused the magazine on the macrobiotic
approach to cancer and other degenerative diseases, on peace
and social justice, and other problems of society. Later, Lenny
Jacobs took control of the magazine. He had been a pioneer
of natural baking and helped us set up the restaurants
downtown.

Year by year, our educational activities continued to grow.
More intensive studies began, and elective courses were added.
Karin Stephan, who organized our first seminar in Paris,
taught Iyengar yoga. Bo-In Lee arrived from Korea to teach
corrective exercises and Mahayana Buddhism. There was
also an Aikido studio. Bill Gleason, a student of ours from
the early days in Boston, returned from Japan after studying
the martial arts for ten years and set up a dōjō next to the
Kushi Institute. Though not directly connected with the K.I.,
it attracted many students.

Teacher certification started. A review board was set up to
maintain teaching and counseling standards. A cook instructor's
service was established to provide cooking and to teach people
how to set up a macrobiotic kitchen at home. Graduates of
the Kushi Institute went on to establish macrobiotic centers
and natural foods manufacturing and distribution companies
of their own. They also served in schools, hospitals, prisons,
nursing homes, and other institutions, influencing dietary
guidelines and bringing a new awareness of health and happiness to thousands of people. As demand increased, with our
associates we set up new Kushi Institutes in Amsterdam,
Antwerp, Florence, Lisbon, Barcelona, Switzerland, and
France.

Our Mountain Retreat in Becket

In Brookline, we soon began to outgrow our school's new space. After a long search, we found a nice property in the Fischer Hill area of town, not far from our home. It was the former site of Cardinal Cushing Junior College. Our home on Buckminster Road was also once owned by Cardinal Cushing College, named after the former archbishop of Boston. In recent years, the Catholic Church's activities had declined, and some of its assets were being sold. Just as Christianity spread through Europe on the sites of former temples and shrines, some friends observed that macrobiotics was succeeding modern religion.

We liked the new site in Brookline very much, but some local residents objected to our moving there. They had opposed the Catholics too, as well as several other religious and charitable organizations which considered moving in. It was clear that they did not object so much to macrobiotics as they were worried about the influx of people and traffic into their neighborhood. We decided to look elsewhere. After a lengthy search, we settled on Becket. Becket proved to be an ideal natural setting for our educational activities. The Franciscans left a calm, peaceful vibration in the buildings and grounds that many visitors have observed. The church fathers themselves were very pleased that their facility would continue to be used to further human health and happiness. Old Father Crispine, the monastery's sole surviving priest, stayed on for awhile. He started eating macrobiotically and experienced more vitality and his arthritis started to go away.

The curriculum at the Kushi Institute was divided into three levels: personal, social, and planetary. The first introduced yin and yang and taught students how to see and improve their own health and happiness. The second level dealt with the health and welfare of the family, community, and nation. The third level focused on problems of world peace, the challenge of biotechnology, new energy sources, and other global events. In the summer and autumn, we began to hold Level

III of the K.I. in Becket. Students found the change from Boston refreshing. In addition to enjoying the beautiful natural environment, they were able to live, cook, and eat together for the first time on a daily basis, developing closer ties and friendships.

In addition to K.I. programs, my husband started spiritual training seminars at Becket, and I began offering advanced cooking intensives. Along with programs offered by our associates, teachers conferences, meetings of the North American Macrobiotic Congress, and other special events, Becket is now an active center for ongoing education year around. Many friends have moved to the area. About half-way between New York and Boston, the Berkshire region is an active cultural and artistic center. In the summer, the Boston Symphony Orchestra gives concerts at Tanglewood in nearby Lenox. The Kripalu Ashram is also located there. Under the guidance of Amrit Desai, a community of several hundred yoga students became macrobiotic and cooperate with us in joint activities.

In Stockbridge, about a half hour's drive from Becket, are other artistic and cultural attractions, including a Shakespeare theater and Ghinga Japanese Macrobiotic Restaurant. *Gingha* means "Silver Stream." This is the Japanese expression for the ribbon of stars in the Milky Way. The Milky Way is associated with an old folk tale about two heavenly lovers. Once upon a time, a young cowherd and fair maiden weaver became so devoted to each other that they neglected their duties and were allowed to see each other only once a year. Every July 15, people in the Far East observe the Star Festival. They pray for clear skies so that the celestial couple can cross over the bridge of silver stars and be reunited. If it is rainy or cloudy, they must wait till the next year for another opportunity to meet. Lafcadio Hearn preserves this legend in his book, *The Romance of the Milky Way*.

Ghinga opened in Stockbridge's old railroad depot on the property of our friends Terrence and Lori Hill, a famous movie actor and producer and his wife. A train still lets people out on the platform. Passengers sometimes come in the back door of the beautifully remodeled station, mistaking the sushi bar for the ticket counter. Ghinga's Japanese chefs specialize in sushi, and it has become one of the most famous restaurants in the Berkshires. In Becket itself, Summit Point, a small, home-style macrobiotic restaurant, opened in an old deer-hunting lodge now shared with a macrobiotic bakery. In the nearby town of Lee, Aveline's, a natural foods store named after me, opened to provide the Berkshire region with good quality food. In North Conway, Christian and Gaelea Elwell, two of our students, had already started the South River Miso Company. It is one of America's pioneer miso-making companies, providing wonderful miso to natural foods stores around the country. In Washington, my sister Yōko and her husband Charles make amazake and mochi under the Kendall Foods label. There are also several large tofu and tempeh companies in the area started by students or friends influenced by our teachings. In Pittsfield, Springfield, and other neighboring communities, our associates have started public education and cooking classes.

The Future of Macrobiotics

In Boston, our activities continue to expand. Everything is now under the direction of the Kushi Foundation, which coordinates the Kushi Institute, *East West Journal*, dietary and way of life counseling, and other programs and events including our foreign seminars. Our main program for the general public is the two-day Way of Life seminar. We have found that unless people actually see the food being prepared, they have a hard time implementing the dietary guidelines. The Way of Life seminar provides a basic introduction to macrobiotics, including beginning cooking classes, meals and an opportunity to share experiences with other participants, and a personal educational interview with my husband or senior teacher. The Way of Life program has become very popular, attracting hundreds of people from across the country every month.

We also have a training program for physicians, nurses,

and other medical professionals. They come from clinics, hospitals, and medical schools to study with us. Dr. Marc van Cauwenberghe directs our educational counseling services and referrals to medical associates. As a young doctor in Belgium, he became inspired by George Ohsawa's writings. He came to Boston with his brother and several other friends to study with us. He is one of the most inspiring teachers of macrobiotics today.

In recent years, a lot of our energy has gone into macrobiotic publishing. For years, my husband's lectures and articles were published in small booklets or magazines mimeographed or printed by his students. These circulated hand to hand. Tao Books in Boston brought out some of this material but later went out of business. In the early 1970s, the *East West Journal* introduced Michio's ideas to a wider audience, and the East West Foundation began publishing *The Order of the Universe*, *Seminar Study Reports*, and several small books.

In 1977, Michio's first major work, *The Book of Macrobiotics*, was brought out by Japan Publications and distributed by Kodansha through Harper & Row. Dozens of other books followed, including my first cookbook, *How to Cook with Miso*. Macrobiotics now accounts for nearly one half of Japan Publication's new titles in English each year. Iwao Yoshizaki, the president of Japan Publications in Tokyo, and Yoshiro Fujiwara, director of the company's American operations in New York, have become warm friends, and my husband and I look forward to their visits to Boston each spring and fall. Mr. Yoshizaki was born in 1923, the Year of the Boar, the same year as me, and has a bold, imaginative outlook. However, his wild boar temperament, unlike mine, has been refined by devotion to classical music, especially Bach. At the annual Frankfurt Book Fair in Germany, he always throws a big party and invites a macrobiotic author to speak at the Japanese restaurant in Goethe House. Thanks to his efforts, macrobiotic literature is now available all over the world.

In 1983, *The Cancer-Prevention Diet*, Michio's first book for a major American publisher, came out. Alex Jack helped him

write it for St. Martin's Press in New York, and it was translated into seven languages. Alex also helped me with my
cookbook, *Aveline Kushi's Complete Guide to Macrobiotic Cooking
for Health, Harmony, and Peace*. Each chapter was prefaced by
one of my pen and ink drawings of life growing up in Yokota
and by haiku written by my pupils in Maki during the war.

There have been many other wonderful macrobiotic books,
including *Recalled by Life* by Dr. Anthony Sattilaro and Tom
Monte, *Macrobiotics: Yesterday and Today* by Ron Kotzsch,
The Way of Life: Macrobiotics and the Spirit of Christianity
by Rev. John Ineson, and *Recovery* by Elaine Nussbaum.
Edward and Wendy Esko, two of our senior associates, have
also pioneered in macrobiotic publishing. They have written
and collaborated with us on many lovely cookbooks, children's
books, and anthologies on the future health of society. They
have six healthy, active children of their own, and it is a
miracle that they can find so much time to write, teach, and
counsel. Ed has a special talent for finding new writers and
has helped develop dozens of new projects.

By the mid-1980s, the majority of the people who came to
the Kushi Institute in Brookline were ordinary Americans.
They were housewives, secretaries, salesmen, mechanics,
lawyers, doctors, teachers, and architects. Many of them were
parents or grandparents. They were more likely to live in
Dallas and Kansas City than in Cambridge or Berkeley. They
were interested in preserving traditional family values, not so
much in achieving personal spiritual enlightenment. They
looked to the Bible for inspiration, not the *I Ching* or *Tao Te
Ching*. They were accustomed to using forks and knives, not
chopsticks.

Macrobiotics may appear to have turned into its opposite
in the course of a generation. But for us, what has altered is
not the spirit, only the form. Over the years, our understanding has constantly grown and developed. Society has also
changed. East and West understand each other better. Modern
medicine and holistic health have begun to see each other as
complementary rather than antagonistic. Macrobiotics is uni-

versal. Young and old, rich and poor, male and female, white and black, red and yellow, liberal and conservative, materialist and spiritualist—everyone can benefit from eating well and studying the order of nature.

My husband and I are optimistic about the future. But much remains to be done. The possibility of nuclear war is still great. Genetic engineering and artificial organ replacements offer another threat to twisting the future course of our species' survival. In the future it may become easier to alter the body and mind technologically than heal it with good food, exercise, and self-reflection. When that happens, our basic human quality and spirit will surely decline. Already, test-tube babies, sperm bank fathers, and surrogate mothers are beginning to upset millions of years of past human evolution. These are enormous challenges. My husband has devoted himself tirelessly in recent years to finding peaceful solutions to the problems of war and biotechnology.

Also challenges to macrobiotic education periodically appear. A few years ago, macrobiotics and other holistic health teachers were charged by some doctors with offering worthless remedies to old people worried about their health. Rep. Claude Pepper's Congressional Subcommittee on Aging investigated these complaints and found that they were groundless. His report concluded that the Standard Macrobiotic Diet was completely nutritious and its dietary approach to cancer was similar to that now being followed by all the major medical associations. Meanwhile, the American Dietetic Association mounted a campaign to monopolize nutritional counseling. Legislation was introduced in many states to give only their own members the right to teach nutrition. Naturally, we defended ourselves. Our teachers and friends who had been helped by macrobiotics testified at legislative hearings. Thousands of people signed petitions at natural foods stores and wrote and called their elected officials. Lawyers and clergymen rallied behind our constitutional right to teach, speak, and assemble. The A.D.A. was defeated in many states. In Massachusetts, the governor issued an annual proclamation proclaiming Natural Health and Nutrition Awareness Month, singling out macrobiotics for its contribution to public health.

Still other obstacles remain to be overcome. Organic farming is still only a small fraction of total modern agriculture. Also for many years, the U.S. Department of Agriculture would not recognize tofu, tempeh, and other vegetable-quality foods as suitable sources of protein. This meant that public schools, hospitals, and other institutions could not use federal funds to purchase these foods for their meal programs. Sometimes the restrictions would be lifted when a new administration, or a new agriculture secretary, came into office. Though weakened by the McGovern Report and the trend toward a low-fat diet, the influence of the dairy and cattlemen's lobby remains strong. So long as budget problems continue in Washington, funding natural foods programs may remain in jeopardy.

Then at the local and state levels, there are numerous ordinances, restrictions, and zoning laws that favor highly processed commercial foods. Again, tempeh, natto, and other soy foods are particularly vulnerable. There is much work that remains to be done to educate consumers, store owners, and government workers and protect the quality of natural foods. The whole foods movement itself has grown fat and lazy over the years. Instead of principle, profit now generally leads. The dream, poetry, and passion that inspired Erewhon, Chico-San, and the other early pioneers are practically nowhere to be found.

Still, America remains the leader in the world today. If we can peacefully change America, we can change the whole world. Looking back on what has been accomplished in just twenty brief years, it is really amazing. When we started, no one made any connection between food and health. The medical and scientific associations thought we were crazy. Now everyone is aware of natural foods. The American Heart Association, the American Cancer Society, and other medical groups have all issued dietary guidelines similar to those given by my husband in lectures and articles decades ago. Their recommended menus now include foods like brown rice, millet, lentils, tofu, whole grain bread, and plenty of fresh vegetables and fruit.

Eating well and restoring physical health is only the beginning of our peaceful revolution. The next step is understanding the connection between what we eat and how we feel. At the social level, men and women will start to come back together as their eating harmonizes. Families will reunite. Young people will be more respectful of their elders and want to learn from them. Old people will be more sympathetic with the problems of the young and share their wisdom and insight. Schools will once again become places of genuine study. Delinquency and crime will diminish. Communities will prosper.

Finally, at the international level, nations of the world will come together and form one planetary commonwealth. Returning to organic and natural agriculture will produce tremendous benefits. The earth's environment will purify itself. Use of land for growing grain and vegetables instead of cattle will provide food in plenty for everyone. It will also enable millions of families uprooted from the soil to return to the land from urban slums and factories. Internationally, there will be less competition for scarce natural resources. Now a huge percentage of the world's oil goes into chemical agriculture, fuel for short automobile trips to the supermarket, synthetic clothing and materials, and other unnecessary or artificial products. Directly or indirectly, changing our way of eating will have limitless benefits for the future health and happiness of our planet.

As natural food penetrates national borders, the conflicts and divisions that separate modern people will decrease. As people around the world eat in the same way, they will begin to think alike. They will see each other as brothers and sisters rather than as enemies. They will gradually get rid of nuclear weapons and other instruments of war. Nations of the world will form a world federation limiting their sovereignty. The world government will be more like a public service or educational body rather than an enforcement or judicial organization. A council of elders—including mothers, fathers, teachers, farmers, artists, children, and others with rich, deep life experience—will guide humanity into a new era of peace.

Our Macrobiotic Congresses which have begun to meet in Europe, North America, the Caribbean, and Middle East are the embryo of future society. Of course, it may be many years before they are mature and strong enough to really inspire and lead society. But it is humanity's last best hope. In the Berkshire area, my husband and I hope to create an open community that can serve as a creative model for the future. In addition to our current activities, we would like to establish there a children's school, a theater for Noh and other traditional drama, and a shrine for world peace. We hope that friends who share our dream will come and build homes on the land or settle in Becket or nearby towns.

Last year, Masanobu Fukuoka, the Japanese farmer and author of *The One-Straw Revolution*, came to Becket to teach natural agriculture. Organic farmers from all over New England came to hear him. He inspired us to try simple, natural methods of farming that have existed for thousands of years and may have formed the foundation for an age when the world was one. It was like seeing Sontoku Ninomiya or other sages from the fabled past. Tears streamed down my face when I heard him talk about his trip to Africa and his proposal for the air forces of the world to drop seeds rather than bombs on the famine-stricken land.

The next day the group met in the garden behind the Kushi Institute dormitory. Mr. Fukuoka explained that the first step in transforming the soil back to its original, fertile condition was to sow daikon seeds everywhere. They grow easily and their long roots help break up the soil.

"This is all very well in theory," someone commented, "but isn't it unecological to transplant long white radish and other Oriental foods to the West?"

"Daikon is not really Eastern," Mr. Fukuoka chuckled in reply. "Yesterday I was walking around and discovered wild daikon growing in the fields and woods. It was native to both hemispheres before they separated in antiquity. The Indians once may have used it. Daikon has just never been domesticated here as it has in the East."

The story is a perfect parable of our times. So many of our difficulties arise from our own misconceptions. To the infinite Order of the Universe, there is no East or West. If only we had eyes to see it, the Kingdom of God, or One Peaceful World, is all around us.

15: An Obi Floating in a Stream

The mind for truth
Begins, like a stream, shallow
At first, but then
Adds more and more depth
While gaining greater clarity.
—Saigyō

WHEN I STUDIED yin and yang at George Ohsawa's school, I could really understand Ninomiya Sontoku's teachings about learning from "the Book of Nature." In the past, I studied many classics and the Bible and relied on them for daily guidance. By watching how everything moves—the stars, nature, animals, people—I began to sense directly the underlying rhythm of life. When I started to teach cooking, my understanding of food as energy developed. I started to see that everything is related, not just physically, but emotionally and spiritually. In the beginning, I used yin and yang in a simple way. Over the years, my understanding has deepened. I experience more variation, connection, and balance.

My view of time and space has also changed. I feel I now have a more comprehensive view than before. I have come to see that past and present are the same. Even if we think we know people presently, they are not much different from people in times past. When I hear about Ninomiya or Kukai, it's the same as if they were alive today. They are as real to me as my family and friends. Sometimes I really question what is past and what is present. As I grow older, death and the future world approach closer. There is not so much difference between this world and the next world. To enter the future world takes only an instant. In western Massachusetts recently, I was driving and my car suddenly swerved on a mountain road and turned over. Fortunately, no one was injured. In time and distance, the next world is closer than Tokyo or Paris. We are within the next world all the time. I have started to think more that way and understand history and the future as one. Like a braid of hair, I begin to see eternal life as an endless meeting and parting of grasses, flowers, clouds, mountains, and people.

At the Kushi Institute, the study of Nine Star Ki has become very popular. This is a form of Far Eastern numerology that can be used to see our destiny. From childhood we knew elements of this system much as Western children know the signs of the zodiac. My husband and I have read many books on the subject and used Nine Star Ki to understand our own characters and personalities, as well as that of our family and friends. In essence, it is the study of moving energy and our relation to the universe. Without really deep understanding, Nine Star Ki sometimes gives only a conceptual, superficial, misguided view of life. We need a more practical, flexible way to see. Although this teaching is highly recommended for understanding the Order of the Universe, it is still not as direct as the way of eating. Unless we are chewing our food thoroughly, no system of prophecy will work very well.

For almost forty years, my husband and I have been repeating the same things to our students. Sometimes I marvel that we don't get tired. Everywhere we go, we say the same thing, show people how to make miso soup and prepare brown rice in the same way, and reply to people's questions in the same broken English. On the surface it looks like nothing changes. But for ourselves, it is never the same. There are always slight changes, modifications, or adjustments to be made. Our understanding constantly grows.

Lately, I discovered the teachings of Nanboku Mizuno. He was born in Japan about 1757 and died about 1835. Nanboku means "North South." He was a physiognomist and devoted his whole life to teaching about food. He worked as an attendant at the public baths and mastered the art of visual diagnosis. He said that food changes into life and that the quality and quantity of food we take almost entirely controls our destiny.

I was astonished. He was saying the exact same things two hundred years ago that my husband and I have been learning to understand more deeply. However, in Mizuno's day, there was no processed food. Instead of quality, he focuses more on quantity. He teaches that too much food can be as harmful as poor quality food. Once you learn to control the quantity of your intake, your whole life changes for the better. You give up excess pounds, excess feelings, excess thoughts. I had learned this with my chanting.

Also at Becket, during spiritual training seminars, we observe a brown rice fast. We eat only rice for four or five days, supplemented with a little miso soup and condiments, and chew each mouthful 150 times. It's amazing how much energy such simple food gives. If you really chew well, you feel satisfied with just one bowl of rice. You begin to realize how much we take in that we don't really need.

This then is the heart of our teaching. Except for slight changes of time and place, my husband and I have arrived at the same place as those who came before us. The end is the beginning, the beginning is the end. All is one. This is the essence of the essence of macrobiotics.

The seeds that Michio and I have spread are the same seeds of joy and love that have always been spread. Countless generations have preceded us, and if we are successful, countless generations shall follow. We really have nothing new to offer. The seeds we scatter blow and go everythere. We don't know where the next one will land, take root, and germinate. Nobody knows what to expect in life. The spirit of true teachings repeats endlessly over thousands and thousands of years. The seeds that we have planted could blossom into a very different kind of world. No one knows for sure.

I hope that our children, students, and friends around the world can grow, adapt, perfect their understanding, and find

314

their own way. Along with my husband, I am content just to have put down beautiful, steady, and possibly deep roots. Eden, Paradise, Utopia, Erewhon, One Peaceful World, Earth—by whatever name, a world of natural beauty and peace is all around us if only we could see it. It's up to God now whether our dream will be realized.

Closing the Circle

Many times people ask if I'm homesick. I tell them, "Not really. The mountains and rivers, the rice fields and wild grasses of Izumo are always living in my heart. Whenever I walk, I have only to close my eyes and remember them deep in my heart. That's why I never feel far away."

When I first went back to Japan after twenty years in America, I was shocked at how much the nation had changed. Even in the countryside, hydroelectric lines, Coke machines, gravel pits, and other evidence of modern civilization was everywhere. For years, I had seen billboards and neon signs around the world for Sanyo, Hitachi, Mazda, Sony, Nissan, and Honda. It was strange seeing them now in Japan.

In Yokota, my hometown, I was saddened to see that chemical farming was a way of life. The farmers wore heavy masks and rubber boots in the fields when they sprayed. The little fishes, grasses, and flowers that once grew amid the grain had all disappeared. Before, the rice fields used to be more naturally shaped, following the contours of the land. Now they are primarily square and rectangular. In other areas, rice fields have been replaced by golf courses, shopping centers, and airports. Thousands of years of traditional organic, natural farming practices in Japan had vanished in the twinkling of an eye. Truly, the great eight-headed dragon of the mountain had reawakened.

Since I left home, Yokota has nearly doubled in size. Its population is now nine thousand. Small industry has come to the valley. One of the main businesses in town is a factory that makes ice cube machines, for export mainly to the United

States. In the next village over, there is a cement factory that has eaten into half the mountain. In Yakawa, near the remote village over the mountains where I once taught, a spring water business has started, one of the first in Japan. The water is used primarily to mix with Scotch. Scotch and whiskey have replaced sake as Japan's favorite drink.

Meat and dairy food consumption in Japan are now nearly universal. Today everyone in Yokota eats beef and drinks milk. The agricultural college at the edge of town where my brother went to school is now a dairy institute. Many rice fields have been turned into pastureland for dairy cows. A typical dairy farm has ten to twenty cattle, the largest has forty. Every household now has an automobile and many have pick-up trucks. The air is not so pure as before. Wide-screen digital televisions, computers, cordless telephones, and all the other conveniences of modern life have come to Yokota.

There used to be a small stream in front of my family's house. Now it is paved over, and there is a busy road. A few doors down is a vending machine that sells ice cream. The old church is still standing, but fewer people attend than before. The beautiful bell in the steeple has been replaced by electronic chimes.

The diseases and disorders of modern civilization have accompanied these changes. When I was little, cancer and heart disease were unknown. Now they are among the leading causes of death in Yokota. The town spends $4 to $6 million a year on medical care. Twenty percent of this amount is subsidized by the government. Taxes are high, and the village is going broke. Everyone is also concerned about the educational system. As elsewhere in Japan, students are pushed relentlessly to compete in the nationwide college entrance exams. Those who score well get admitted to the top schools, automatically go on to the biggest companies, and are guaranteed a life of wealth and status. Students who fail the exams sometimes commit suicide, and such tragedies have become a routine part of modern life in Japan. In Yokota, I was saddened to hear that one high school girl recently took her own life. Violence, delinquency, and crime are also appearing. Farmers are keeping their doors closed for the first time.

My old classmates, teachers, students, and friends have all been affected by these changes. Mitsuko Yodono, who lived in town and introduced me to macrobiotics, died of breast cancer. She had moved to Brazil and visited us once in Boston. I regretted that my husband and I were unable to help her at that time. In Kyoto, I met Ken-chan, my childhood playmate. He was the son of Mr. Okazaki, our village leader. We had not seen each other for over thirty years. He told me he has suffered from diabetes for most of this time. He works for a big pharmaceutical company in Kyoto testing monkeys. His biggest worry is protests from animal lovers. Nearly everyone I met was suffering from some illness, family problem, or social conflict.

Japan had turned into its opposite. I guess I should not really have been surprised. The first law of the Order of the Universe is that everything changes. And at their extreme, yin turns to yang, yang turns to yin.

Eventually the pendulum starts to swing the other way. On a subsequent visit to Yokota, I met a bright young man. His name was Junichi Sato, and he was about thirty years old. He had been a rice farmer, cultivating his family fields like generations of ancestors before him. Recently he entered village politics and won election to town council. With a small group of other officials, he decides matters relating to local agriculture, education, social services, culture and the arts.

During my visit, I spoke to a few friends and townspeople about my activities. One of the people who came to my talk was Mr. Sato. Macrobiotics' traditional, commonsense view of life appealed to him, and he immediately changed his way of eating.

Later that year, he came to America to visit the Kushi Institute. Back home, Mr. Sato organized a small macrobiotic club in Yokota. There are now several dozen friends eating brown rice, miso soup, and other traditional foods in my home town.

As a farmer, parent, and town official, Mr. Sato is particularly concerned with the effects of modern agriculture and industry. Izumo's beautiful wildlife and environment are dying. Wilderness areas are vanishing, and everywhere developers are using chemicals. Bears, foxes, badgers, rabbits, rats, and snakes are coming down from the mountains into the valleys as their natural homes are destroyed. Loggers have come in and cut down large stands of oaks and maples, leaving less profitable evergreens. Some of these trees are said to have been planted in ancient times and figure in stories in the *Kojiki*. Leaving only one kind of tree growing creates poor soil, water, and mineral conditions throughout the forest. Birds will no longer nest in the trees. Wild boars have come back in the countryside and are eating the farmers' bamboo. The palm trees have all died from insects, and pine moths are killing the pines. The fish in the streams have thinned. Even the tea bushes growing on the side of the hills yield leaves giving a funny taste.

Mr. Sato and his associates have started to alert people to the loss of their beautiful homeland. Thanks to their efforts, some reforestation programs have started. A mixture of deciduous and evergreen trees has been planted. Wildlife is beginning to come back.

Closer to home, the small macrobiotic community in Yokota has begun to educate people about food and health. Organically grown brown rice, other grains and beans, traditionally made miso, tamari soy sauce, and other nourishing foods are now available. Many of the town's old people remember the foods they ate growing up. They can see clearly how weak the younger generation is in comparison. They have started to think about food and its relation to sickness and to the wild behavior of children in schools.

The biggest opposition to macrobiotics has come over the issue of dairy food. Dairy farming is now the biggest food industry in the valley. Dairy farmers, merchants, doctors, and others influenced by modern thought are opposed to anything that calls into question the value of milk, cheese, and ice cream.

Mr. Sato, however, is optimistic. He thinks it will take

about five years to change the village. He arranged for my husband and me to meet with the mayor of Yokota and other leading citizens to explain our teachings. One new friend who became macrobiotic is a young dairy farmer. He says that as soon as possible he would like to convert back to rice or some other crop for the health and happiness of his family and the valley. In Maki, over the mountains, one of my former pupils, now a mother herself, said she would like to sell one of her baby cows and use the money to come visit the Kushi Institute in Boston.

After Mr. Sato returned from the United States, the macrobiotic community in Yokota decided to become a sister city with Becket. In the future, they hope young people from Japan and America will go back and forth, visiting each other's regions and helping in farming, natural food production, and traditional arts and crafts. I have been very moved by the earnestness and energy shown by the young people of my home country. The passion, poetry, and dream that George Ohsawa's students had in Hiyoshi and that our early students had in Boston are now alive in them. Like the prisoners we visited in Portugal and the friends with AIDS in New York, they are true macrobiotic revolutionaries.

I am confident that they will be able to subdue the reawakened dragon of the mountain. Like a Noh drama, modern life in Izumo and everywhere around the world has been sorrowful. But in the end, disorder is overcome by strength of spirit and gentle means such as prayer, chanting, and cooking with love. The demons are dispersed, and peace returns.

Student-Teacher Reunion

In Okazaki, a city famous as the home of Hatcho miso, I met Mr. Tanaka, my old college teacher. Our correspondence had resumed since he wrote the foreword to my students' book of haiku. I had seen him several times on speaking tours of Japan, but we didn't have much chance to visit.

We met at a coffee shop on top of a large hotel. It looked

out over the the lovely winding rivers and rolling hills of the region. The shōgun who founded the Tokugawa era had once lived in Okazaki, but his castle couldn't have had such a spectacular view. I noticed Mr. Tanaka's strong constitution. His eyebrows were thick and long, and he had big ears and hands, traditional signs of longevity. His hair was still black with flecks of silver. He was immaculately dressed in a black pinstripe suit and tie with brown and red stripes.

Mr. Tanaka had retired from teaching but was still active promoting the ideals of Sontoku Ninomiya, the peasant sage. He told me there were thirty Hōtoku "Return to Gratitude" clubs devoted to his philosophy. As he talked, I noticed the same expression and gentle hand movements he made years ago in class to illustrate a point.

"Japanese society today is very bad for children," he observed softly, his voice breaking. "There is too much pressure. Children come home after school with heavy shoulders. All they do is study. They've lost their freedom and happiness. They've lost their true nature. They watch TV, but they are not really enjoying themselves. Instead of a ten-minute break, give them twenty. Then their study will improve. They need more free time."

He told me his own grandson lives nearby. But the boy studies until 6 P.M. and they have no time to talk. He said that society rewards intelligence and clever thinking, but not creativity.

"Besides study, children today need to develop a real dream or create something in life," he reflected.

The next day, I stopped at his house to say goodbye. In the garden, amid the bonsai trees and wonderful rocks, Mr. Tanaka showed me a small statue to his students that he had put up. He told me that our class in Hamada was his first class, and he had always regarded it as special. He said that he learned education from us. The inscription on the stone read:

If you just look, they are my children,

If you look very well, they took care of me.
I grew because of them.

On this visit, I also met some of my old classmates and
students. I had not seen many of them since World War II.
They were all so surprised at the course my life had taken.
They couldn't believe I was teaching cooking. They said they
thought I would become a star gymnast or a martial artist.
In Yokota, Dr. Fujiwara, who had nursed me back to health,
gave me the little book of poems I had written on my sick
bed. He had kept them all these years.

In Hamamatsu, I went to visit Oritaro Shimizu, who paid
for my trip to America. He and his wife were now in their
mid-nineties. Mr. Shimizu had enormous ears that lay flat
to the sides of his head like a Buddha. His head was bald or
completely shaved like a monk. Long whispy white and black
eyebrows framed bright, sparkling eyes. He punctuated his
conversation with vigorous gestures of his thick fingers.

Before the war, Mr. Shimizu and his family owned big silk
and cotton weaving mills. They lost everything in the bombing. From the ashes, Mr. Shimizu started to rebuild his life
and fortune. After the war, he started farming. His son went to
Tokyo and studied macrobiotics. When George Ohsawa introduced us, Mr. Shimizu said he believed in world government
and the plan to send twelve ambassadors of peace around the
world, including Michio and myself. Although he had no
money, he said he would see what he could do. He borrowed
the funds for my trip to America from neighboring rice
farmers.

Later, Mr. Shimizu donated part of his property to a small
motorcycle company. It's name was Honda. He and his wife
now live in a modest house next to Honda's headquarters.
In addition to his fabric factories and mills which have been
rebuilt, Mr. Shimizu has extensive overseas interests. He
is chairman of Yaohan with six supermarkets in Los
Angeles, New Jersey, Costa Rica, and Malaysia. He has
become a renowned industrialist, philanthropist, and elder

statesman. People from all over Japan come to him for sage advice.

Mr. Shimizu attributes a good deal of his success and vitality to his diet, which is essentially macrobiotic. He says that he has continued to eat brown rice. Next door he showed us a small kitchen in the Honda plant where he is manu-facturing dried brown rice cakes for export through his food stores. He is also active in the Sei Cho No Ie, one of the new religions.

At his house, Mr. Shimizu showed us scrolls that he was making. They were fan-shaped and stacked high against the wall. There were enough for each of his ten children and forty-eight grandchildren and great-grandchildren. After dipping their hands in red ink, he and his wife each make a palm print on the scroll. Then he inscribes a poem on the gold-leaf back-ground in a firm, bold hand.

"My wife is very simple," he told us with smiling eyes. "She has always followed my lead. God is pleased with her. Eternally we are peaceful. We are making these scrolls for our children and grandchildren. If we left them our fortune, they would become spoiled. Instead we will just leave these poems."

When it was time for my husband and me to go, Mr. Shimizu gave us one of the scrolls.

Return to Hiyoshi

In Tokyo, I had a reunion with several friends from George Ohsawa's dormitory. Several of them were still teaching macrobiotics, like Abe and Aida Nakamura who were visiting from Germany where they have lived for the last thirty years. Others like Uka Onoda (Bernadette), the sculptress, had incorporated the teachings into their career. But some had gone off the diet and suffered as a result.

One of the men who came to our reunion was Yoshitaro Kaneko. I recognized him as Balzac, the tall, dapper young man whom I had fished from Shinjuku Station. He was much heavier now, with somewhat of a paunch. He told me that he had gone on to a career in photography and helped pioneer the strobe light. His company was very famous. He had a wife and two children. Over the years, he had strayed from macrobiotics. Then he found that he had colon cancer. He started eating brown rice again. He started chewing each bite of food two hundred times. He started singing a happy song before every meal. Gradually he recovered.

Once you experience or study macrobiotics, you can't escape. If you don't practice well and get sick, at least in your mind food and health are always associated. I was very happy to hear of Balzac's recovery. He wrote up his experience in a macrobiotic journal in Tokyo and is now helping Lima Ohsawa in her activities.

Following our reunion, several of us went to Hiyoshi to see the site of the old Maison Ignoramus. From Tokyo it is only about a half-hour's ride. Passing through Shinjuku Station, memories of selling the World Government newspaper on the platform flooded my mind. I thought of Garry Davis, the young world citizen whose adventures were chronicled in the newspaper. Just recently, after more than thirty years, my husband and I had connected with him. He was still traveling everywhere without a passport and braving jail for being a free man. We invited Garry to speak at the Kushi Institute and our summer camp, and he started to incorporate macrobiotics into his world government philosophy.

From the Hiyoshi train station, we walked up the little main street. There were many changes, but the shops were still modest. Some stocked fresh vegetables. I noticed the broccoli as we passed. In the old days, it was unknown. I first had broccoli in New York. At the police station, we turned right. A few blocks ahead was the location of George Ohsawa's old school. As we approached it, I felt a sense of anticipation as I had the first early morning when I arrived from Izumo. Would it even be there? Perhaps it had been turned into a golf course.

My heart fluttered as I recognized the boys' dormitory

behind the hedge. Of course, the big World Government sign on top of the building had long been taken down. Turning the corner, I caught a glimpse of the white house next door. It was still there! My heart was beating rapidly. The small stucco structure was one story then. Now I noticed a second story, and the shutters had been painted brown. The garden was more enclosed than before. Amid the ornamental shrubs and trees, I recognized the gnarled plum tree. It was like an old friend. The bright red camellia flowers looked just the same. The pine tree at the side of the gate still jutted out at an unusual angle. A new stone path had been laid in the garden.

By the front gate, we ran into the current owner. She told us that her parents had bought the house thirty-four years ago. They expanded one end and added a bedroom on the far side. We told her that we had been students here many years ago. The lady said she was aware that there was some kind of young people's school here in the past but didn't know what was being taught. Opening onto the garden was George Ohsawa's old room. Happy memories returned of listening to his lectures. And in the back where the woodshed used to be, I saw the place where I had picked up the axe and earned my nickname.

With tears of joy in our eyes, we walked back to the train station. George Ohsawa had lived here only four years. It was a short time really, but how many lives he had touched. And what had started here had now spread all over the world.

Visit to a Shrine

Wakayama province, in southwestern Honshū, is one of the most beautiful in Japan. At the tip of Kii Peninsula, Kumano juts into the Pacific Ocean, and according to legend, from there holy men traditionally set sail for the Blessed Isles of Kannon, the Bodhisattva of Compassion. My husband, who was born there and whose ancestors lived there for centuries, compares it to an earthly paradise. In Kumano there is a small

shrine that is said to be the oldest in Japan. It is connected to
Izumo, my home province, in a curious way. After subduing
the eight-headed dragon, Susa-no-wo married Kushi-Inada-
Hime. The grandson of the the Wind God and the Wondrous
Princess of the Ricefields settled on the northern coast of
Izumo. He became revered as the symbol of prosperity and
long life and the teacher of medicine. A shrine in his honor
was built in Kumano and another one in Izumo.

In olden days, people from all over Japan came to the
Kumano Shrine to pay their respects. Later, about two thousand years ago, the present Imperial line began, and the new
capital was established in Nara and later Kyoto. Every emperor went to the small Kumano Hongu Shrine to pray and
receive guidance as did the priests of other shrines, including
the famous Ise Shrine. In the Kumano Shrine, a small fire was
made with stones and wood. A flame would be carried back
by visitors to light other sacred fires in shrines and temples
around the land.

On New Year's Day, rulers and officials would bring mochi,
or pounded sweet rice, as a gift to the temple. The guardians
of the Kumano Shrine always greeted them in the same way.
"Your mochi is not so well prepared. Its taste could be
improved. Maybe it should be cooked a little bit longer.
However, considering your efforts and hard work, we can
accept it this year, but next time please do better."

By this, they meant that the lords had not taken care of the
people as well as they could in the year just past. The roads
could be repaired. Taxes could be lowered. Things could be
improved. They must strive harder in the year ahead. Such
was the custom. For thousands of years, this ritual was
observed.

For years, my husband had wanted to visit the Kumano
Shrine in Izumo. Although it was very famous, he and I had
never been there. Finally, on a recent trip to Japan, he had an
opportunity to travel there. He had been in Tokyo lecturing
on the macrobiotic approach to AIDS and cancer. He had
given many interviews to the press and television and coun-

seled many people who beseiged him for guidance in their personal problems. As usual, he didn't have a free moment but really wished to see the Kumano Shrine.

"When I arrived at the Kumano Shrine," Michio later told his students at a spiritual training seminar in Becket, "I finally understood all these years why I wanted to come here. What god is enshrined there? Kushi-Mike-No-Mikoto*, the God of Food and Way of Life. His spirit is there. He is the one who married the Princess of the Rice Fields. I finally understood my destiny. I understood the meaning of my marriage."

When he came to America, my husband was not really following a macrobiotic way of eating. I haven't made any contribution to his character or personality, but over the years I have influenced his diet. In New York, Boston, and capitals around the world, he has stirred up things like the impetuous Wind God of legend. He has taught people new ways of farming, eating, and living harmoniously with nature.

Amid so much activity, I have not always taken proper care of Michio as a wife. But I have provided good food every day and seen that he has maintained his daily health. He might have married someone else, but he would not teach as he does today. He might have come to the view that food is important without my help, but he would have gone in another direction. I have remained a poor country girl, from the deep mountains of Izumo to the mountains of Becket. If I have succeeded at all as his partner in life, it is in accomplishing this. Of that, I am proud. As I concluded in my cookbook, *Aveline Kushi's Complete Guide to Macrobiotic Cooking for Health, Harmony, and Peace:*

> When you have mastered the various elements that go into preparing brown rice—salt, fire, water, pressure, and a calm mind—your family will attain enduring health and happiness. You will have united yin and yang—Kushi Inada-Hime and Susa-no-wo-no-mikoto. The gleaming sword of supreme judgment will stand unveiled to be

---

* One of the names of Susa-no-wo.

passed down through your cooking, your love, and your spirit to generations without end.

"And the Greatest of These . . ."

In his silkscreen shop, my father used to make his own patterns. He was an expert at cutting the cloth, making prints, and dyeing the fabric different colors. Farmers and townspeople would bring him their brocade. He especially liked to inscribe family crests on kimonos. As a little girl, I loved to watch and help him in his work. Some of my happiest memories are at his side in the shop while mother prepared dinner in the kitchen and my brothers and sisters played in the garden. Unfortunately, all the fabric of his that had come down to me had worn out or been lost over the years.

Matsue, the capital of Izumo province, is located up the coastline from the Izumo Shrine. Across from the city's old castle is the Lafcadio Hearn Museum. My son and grandson who were traveling with me took a tour of the museum while I went to meet some old classmates from Teachers' College. Hearn's original manuscripts are displayed in the museum. It is a real treasure house for folk tales, ghost stories, and legends of old Japan. In recent years, Hearn's books have not been so widely read. People today find his stories of communicating with spirits and unusual coincidences too fanciful to believe.

In Hamada, I met my old classmates for lunch at a hotel. We had not seen each other for over forty years. One of my friends, Masu Horaya, handed me a small parcel. I unwrapped it. I was so surprised. Inside was an obi that my father made out of silk years ago. An obi is the wide sash that is used to tie a kimono. It is worn around the hara, the balancing point, the place where creation begins and the flame of life is kept.

My friend told me that there had just been a flood in her house and everything was destroyed except the obi which floated free. The cloth was dyed black and was emblazoned with a pink dragon with spiral motifs. She said she thought

I should have it. I was grateful and thanked her for her
kindness. Then my thoughts naturally turned to my family
and ancestors in the world of spirit. This heaven-sent gift was
another reminder that life is an endless river and that everything changes. Only love endures.

You Are One Seed

All of you are small seeds, seeds of wonder.
Someday you will all become a great tree
And cover the whole sky, casting a cool shadow
To give rest and new energy to tired travelers and
    inspire them to continue their journey.
You will become a great tree like this.

Many children will climb up and play in your branches.
From early morning till sunset flocks of chirping
    birds will perform on your orchestral stage.
Year by year your blossoms will grow giving joy to
    thousands and millions of people.
In the winter, brilliant stars will shine on top of your
    branches.
In autumn, you will dress up gorgeously and cover the
    ground with your golden leaves.
You will become a distant landmark for people passing
    in a faraway field.
You are the seeds of such a great, great tree.

Like seeds that spend the long, long winter below zero
    underground,
The hammer of that strong coldness you are receiving.
The heavy frozen earth presses down on you.
If you just wait patiently, spring will come and your
    seeds will start to sprout.
If you don't sprout and become such a big tree, the heavy
    wind and snow will crack your boughs.
If you don't become such a big tree and continue growing

for a hundred or thousand years and put out strong
branches toward the whole sky, the cold, heavy, strong
hammering you are receiving is not enough.

Totenkhan . . . totenkhan . . . totenkhan . . .
The sound of the strong, severe blacksmith's hammer
which is Heaven and Earth, yin and yang's order.

Dear seeds, dear seeds,
You shall become a great, great tree.
Tiny, tiny jewel seeds,
You are magical seeds,
More wonderful than diamonds and emeralds.
Dear magical seeds,
Quickly sprout out.

Totenkhan . . . totenkhan . . . totenkhan . . .
May your leaves appear quickly.
May your hands and arms stretch out straight
Toward the sky which is endlessly blue.

Dear seeds, dear seeds, magical seeds.
All of you really wonder if you will grow a hundred,
thousand, million times and turn into a great tree and
live for a thousand years with a beautiful canopy of
leaves.
Of you wonder if you will become small, nasty, and
disorderly as a low bush.
That all depends on your will.
This is what you are wondering about.
If you wish to be a great tree, then you need a great,
big hammering.
If you wish to be a small tree, then you need a small
hammering.
Silently, quietly, just receive it.
That alone is enough.
If you escape a big hammering, you will only become
a small, weak, tiny tree.

As human seeds, you have feet.
You are able to escape from those great hammerings or
 jump into them under the big hammer.
Ah! Seeds with feet!

Dear seeds, dear seeds, magical seeds,
Sprout out, sprout out, quickly sprout out.
Stick out your chin, reach out your hands, raise up
 your heads.

—GEORGE OHSAWA
On Saying Farewell to Aveline
and the M. I. Children
July, 1951

*　　　*　　　*

Dear George!
 I wonder whether I have received enough hammering
to be strong.
 My roots in New England may not be deep enough
yet.
 I know that I may not be fully grown.
 I am still a sapling.
 But I have many seeds, which are sprouting. They
will grow much taller than I, just as you had hoped.
 Nearly forty years have passed since I left my country.
 Now I can much more clearly understand and appre-
ciate your poem.
 I will pass on your beautiful words to my children,
grandchildren, all my friends and students.

AVELINE KUSHI
January 24, 1988

Macrobiotic Resources

For information on macrobiotic activities in the United States and abroad, including Aveline Kushi's teaching schedule, please contact:

The Kushi Institute
P.O. Box 1100
Brookline, Mass. 02147
(617) 738–0045

Kushi Foundation Berkshires Center
P.O. Box 7
Becket, Mass. 01223
(413) 623–5742